Nelson Ivan Chavez Mostajo

# GERIATRIC SYNDROMES FOR RESIDENT PHYSICIANS

Nelson Ivan Chavez Mostajo

# GERIATRIC SYNDROMES FOR RESIDENT PHYSICIANS

## Integrating B-Learning in Geriatrics: A New Era in Teaching

ScienciaScripts

Cover image: www.ingimage.com

This book is a translation from the original published under ISBN 978-613-9-40861-0.

Publisher:
Sciencia Scripts
is a trademark of
Dodo Books Indian Ocean Ltd. and OmniScriptum S.R.L publishing group

120 High Road, East Finchley, London, N2 9ED, United Kingdom
Str. Armeneasca 28/1, office 1, Chisinau MD-2012, Republic of Moldova, Europe
Printed at: see last page
**ISBN: 978-620-7-84537-8**

***TEACHING GERIATRIC SYNDROMES TO MEDICAL RESIDENTS THROUGH B-LEARNING***

***INTEGRATING B-LEARNING IN GERIATRFA: A NEW ERA IN EDUCATION***

## PRÔLOGO

It is a pleasure to present this book entitled "Teaching Geriatric Symptoms to Resident Physicians from B-Learning", which focuses on the integration of hybrid learning (B-Learning) in the teaching of geriatrics. This text arises in response to the growing need to adapt medical training to the current and future demands of an ageing population, offering educational tools that combine face-to-face teaching with digital technologies.

Geriatrics, as a branch of medicine, is dedicated to the study and management of diseases affecting the elderly, as well as to the promotion of healthy ageing. In this context, effective and up-to-date teaching of geriatric syndromes becomes crucial in order to train professionals capable of dealing with the complex challenges presented by this stage of life. Geriatric syndromes, such as immobility, drowsiness, urinary incontinence, cognitive impairment, sarcopenia and frailty, represent conditions that significantly affect the quality of life of older adults and require an interdisciplinary and personalised approach.

This book not only presents a comprehensive compendium of theoretical and practical knowledge about these syndromes, but also introduces the B-Learning method as an innovative strategy for medical education. Through this methodology, resident doctors have the opportunity to learn in a flexible and dynamic way, combining the advantages of face-to-face teaching with the possibilities offered by digital tools.

The main objective of this text is to provide resident physicians with a comprehensive and accessible resource that will enable them to develop clinical competencies and critical skills in the management of geriatric syndromes. Through case studies, interactive exercises and multimedia resources, readers will be able to delve deeper into the clinical and ethical aspects of geriatric care, fostering a holistic and humanised understanding of the care of older adults.

I would like to express my gratitude to all the contributors who have made this book possible. Their dedication and commitment to medical education and the well-being of older adults have been instrumental in the creation of this book. It is my hope that this book will serve as a valuable guide and an incentive for resident physicians to continue their medical education. training with enthusiasm and dedication, always in pursuit of excellence in geriatric care.

Finally, I invite readers to explore and make the most of the content and resources presented in this book, in the conviction that lifelong learning and innovative learning are essential to meet the challenges of an ageing population and to improve the quality of life of our elders.

M.Sc Nelson Ivan Chavez Mostajo Cochabamba 31 May 2024

# CHAPTER 1
# INTRODUCTION TO GERIATRICS AND GERONTOLOGY

## 1. Introduction to Geriatrics and Gerontology

Geriatrics and gerontology are disciplines concerned with preventing, delaying and modifying the biological, psychological, social and economic processes associated with ageing. Gerontology studies aspects of ageing and old age throughout the individual's life span, approaching them from a bio-psychosocial perspective (Zarebski, 2021).

Gerontology, defined by the American functionalist Robert Butler, is the science that investigates ageing in all its dimensions. Butler highlighted the importance of studying human ageing as early as the 17th century, focusing on significant contributions from various scientific fields.

The main difference between geriatrics and gerontology is that geriatrics is primarily a care discipline, which integrates techniques, knowledge and skills aimed at the preservation of physical, psychological and social functioning throughout life. Gerontology, on the other hand, not only focuses on the care aspect but also investigates the chronological evolution of all dimensions of the human being.

The aim of geriatrics is to promote an active and healthy old age throughout the life cycle. This discipline focuses on specific problems of old age, such as polypharmacy, diabetes and memory disorders, and on the implementation of new methods of care such as day centres, chronic hospitals and geriatric units (Zarebski, 2021). (Zarebski, 2021).

Research in gerontology encompasses sociological, economic, epidemiological and physiological aspects, with the aim of comprehensively understanding the ageing process. Moreover, this discipline is fundamental to design and improve welfare and care programmes for the elderly population, promoting active and healthy ageing.

### 1.1. Geriatrics and Gerontology: Definition and Coverage

Actions in geriatric medicine are comprehensive and holistic, considering the environment, mental state, co-morbidity, degree of independent and social living, as well as the views of the subject and their non-professional caregivers. The ultimate goal is to achieve that adults over 65 are free of chronic diseases and enjoy a good quality of life. (Mazzini et al., 2023).

The overall goal in geriatrics is disease prevention through health promotion and disease protection, early diagnosis, comprehensive treatment and management of chronic pathology by controlling risk factors. In addition, it seeks to prevent negative consequences on health once the disease has already appeared (Gonzalez-Montalvo et al., 2020).

In the field of public health, Geriatrics and Gerontology focus on the study and care of the elderly as vital components of society. From this approach, the aim is to improve the quality of life of older adults and prevent diseases associated with ageing (Pifia et al., 2022).It is important to note that the increase in the older population has led to significant changes in the disease profile. Most chronic diseases now limit functional capacity, while specific conditions of old age, such as dementia, delirium, diabetes, caesthesia, malnutrition and pressure ulcers, are responsible for the greatest functional impairment in the elderly. Functional impairment in frail elderly people leads to high resource consumption and high resource utilisation.Chronic diseases, many of which are influenced by lifestyle, account for up to 90% of the leading causes of premature death and disease, with the presence of degenerative diseases increasing as well. The ageing process is a stage that all individuals experience and that often limits or complicates the performance of daily activities (Burgos et al., 2023).

### 1.2. Importance and relevance in today's society

The progressive change in family structures affects the forms of care for older people, manifesting itself in various forms of discrimination, both implicit and explicit. This requires professionals to take an active role. The evolution towards what is called the "new family" or "polyhedral family", characterised by a reduction in the number of members, in the birth rate, in the length of intergenerational cohabitation, in the size of dwellings, and changes in the role and location of women, poses dynamic challenges in geriatric care, creating specific demands on health professionals. (Parrales & Molina, 2020) The "geriatricization" of resources, benefits and services has become a palpable reality, not only in the health care field, but also extending to the care of the elderly in all sectors of social activity (Landazabal & Barboza, 2020). (Landazabal & Barboza, 2020) In this context, professionals not only provide care to patients, but must also facilitate and develop promotion, prevention, rehabilitation and social care programmes, efficiently manage needs, take into account the wishes of those concerned, facilitate family participation, know about residential alternatives, and manage economic resources.

Moreover, the growing number of elderly people, who reach old age in heterogeneous physical and psychological conditions, increases the demand for a higher quality of care. The process of population ageing has generated an exponential increase in the geriatric population, affecting the population pyramid as a priority and generating highly specific social and care demands, such as socialisation problems and the need for new benefits and specialised services. Among the demand-side factors, the need for knowledge in gerontology and geriatrics among professionals working in social and/or health care is widely recognised. (Arias et al., 2020) Understanding and adapting services to the specific needs of older adults is fundamental to ensure active and healthy ageing. (Zubiria, 2024; Malan Valente, 2024).

### 1.3. Objectives and benefits of studying Geriatrics and Gerontology

Primary care doctors and nurses acquire specific knowledge to provide older people in their service portfolio with adequate quality care, to plan health promotion programmes, to prevent and avoid complications, to detect early and treat diseases of old age, and to include healthy habits and attitudes.Geriatric specialists, as well as geriatric-trained internists, should receive comprehensive training to enable them to manage the clinically complex and socially unprotected situations of older patients. This includes applying principles of functionality, participation and independence, and assuming an essential role in the processes of assessment, prevention and treatment. In addition, they must contribute, within a multidisciplinary team, to the care of specific groups of patients in highly complex services requiring hospitalisation or gerontological social care. Geriatrics and Gerontology residents, having become familiar with the basic concepts of ageing, will develop critical thinking skills and understand the multifactorial complexity of the ageing process. This knowledge will enable them to deal effectively with the care of older patients, discovering the attractive and challenging aspects of this speciality.

These professionals will also have an in-depth knowledge of the geriatric characteristics of the diagnostic, therapeutic and preventive resources shared with the rest of clinical medicine. Participate in the development of specialised and multidisciplinary medicine for the elderly. They will learn to apply this knowledge in clinical interventions and specific health programmes, and will develop the ability to identify, design and apply research projects that help to resolve the lack of scientific evidence in the geriatric field, focusing on preventive and therapeutic aspects of certain diseases.

## 2. Biological Aspects of Ageing

The ageing process must be understood as a natural, progressive, deleterious and universal phenomenon, as it affects all body systems. Biologically, changes in DNA, gene expression and cell function are observed. In addition, there are alterations in the immune system and in the homeostasis of the organism. It is crucial to consider various biological aspects that influence this process, such as the accumulation of cellular damage and the decrease in the regenerative capacity of tissues, which are key factors in ageing (Ramfrez, 2023). (Ramfrez, 2023).

Chronic inflammation and oxidative stress also play significant roles in this process. In addition, immunosenescence, or ageing of the immune system, increases vulnerability to various diseases. Hormonal changes are equally impactful, contributing to the onset of age-related diseases and decreased functional capacity. (Ramfrez, 2023)

The first phase of ageing marks the transition from the period of postnatal development - in which the organism increases in size and weight - to a period of stagnation in which growth ceases. From this point, organ size is maintained by the growth of cells, which eventually enter the G0 phase of the cell cycle, ceasing division and reaching a constant size. These cells adapt to functional demands through a local feedback system that controls their growth. Over time, the cells may increase in size, sometimes pathologically, until they reach a point of of nuclear stasis, at which point cell division is halted due to the presence of a massive amount of sephialytic markers (CISNEROS, 2021).Subsequently, specific sequences of morphological alterations can be observed in the nucleus that affect markers of cellular ageing and cell functionality. These changes include alterations in gene expression and the accumulation of DNA damage, which contribute to the deterioration of cellular homeostasis and the development of age-related diseases. (CISNEROS, 2021)

## 2.1. Physiological and anatomical changes in the ageing process

The ageing process is characterised by a series of physiological and anatomical changes that affect various body systems. These changes include alterations in chromatin, DNA methylation, histone modifications and RNA profiles that have profound implications for cellular functioning (Kanasi et al., 2016).

In the brain, ageing leads to morphological changes in cortical thickness, surface area and grey matter volume, reflecting specific histological changes during the ageing process (Lemaître et al., 2012). Age-related alterations in swallowing function, influenced by anatomical and physiological changes in the head and neck, increase the risk of dysphagia in older adults (Ney et al., 2009). In addition, significant deviations from linearity are observed in brain structure, indicative of age-related changes in areas such as the cerebral cortex and diencephalon (Jernigan et al., 1991).

In the musculoskeletal system, ageing can lead to anatomical variations and bone changes, especially in the lumbosacroiliac region of the spine (Scilimati et al., 2022). Physiological and anatomical changes in the pelvic floor during pregnancy and postpartum may affect pelvic organ support and continence (Gondim et al., 2022).

Ageing also involves changes in cellular homeostatic mechanisms, reduction in organ mass and decrease in the functional reserve of body systems (Nigam et al., 2012). These alterations are a consequence of reduced physical activity and the ageing process itself (Amarya et al., 2018). Chronic patients present a complexity that increases with age, accumulating problems such as memory impairment, gait difficulties, hearing and vision loss, increasing their vulnerability to acute illness.

In the global assessment of geriatric patients, it is essential to consider aspects such as functional status and autonomy, psychological, emotional and motivational status, social environment, quality of life and social roles, socio-economic status, family integration, dependency, adaptation and social realisation (Gonzalez-Montalvo et al., 2020). The purpose of this assessment is to categorise, identify, assess and make decisions about actions to be taken, including treatment and follow-up.

The elderly population is diverse in terms of health and diseases. The clinical pathophysiological and clinical-therapeutic peculiarities in terms of response and evolution may vary significantly from one elderly patient to another, due to the ageing process, multiple associated chronic diseases and their treatments, as well as different personal background and environmental factors (Reyna et al., 2021).

In conclusion, ageing manifests itself through a multitude of physiological and anatomical changes in various body systems. Understanding these alterations is crucial for addressing age-related health problems and developing specific interventions to promote healthy ageing.

## 2.2. Biological and non-biological theories of ageing

Considered as mechanical theorists (Cartesian concept), they assume ageing as a process that inexorably leads to deterioration and loss of function, presenting a view of the elderly as weak and passive individuals. (Yungplut, 2024).

However, ageing is nowadays conceived with a more dynamic and complex nuance involving many factors, called biological ageing theories.

Following Aristotle's criteria, it was not until the 19th century that ageing was considered as a possible study. From the beginning of biological knowledge and throughout the Middle Ages and the Modern Age, ageing was considered to occur as a consequence of the heat generated in the body and which was eventually consumed. It was from the beginning of the 19th century, after centuries of considering that man hardly changed in his years, and that it was very easy to be a wise old person, that many hypotheses and hypotheses began to be put forward. research related to embryonic growth, development and ageing (Garcfa Montes de Oca & en Estomatologfa).

Theories of human ageing are classified into two groups, according to the discipline that has generated them: biological and extrabiological. Historically, biology has explained ageing on the basis of the changes that occur in the organism over the years. However, since the mid-20th century, the multicultural nature of society and the growing interest in older adults have demonstrated the need to review the conception of ageing from different perspectives, such as epidemiology, psychology and sociology. (LA)(Grande Aranda, 2024).

## 2.3. Prevention and management of common diseases in old age

Disease prevention in old age requires a thorough understanding of the molecular mechanisms underlying ageing and age-related pathologies. A key factor is chronic inflammation, characterised by upregulation of proinflammatory mediators due to redox imbalance, which plays an important role in ageing and associated diseases (Chung et al., 2009). Furthermore, low-grade chronic inflammation, perpetuated by dietary factors, can promote conditions such as obesity and osteoporosis, highlighting the importance of lifestyle interventions for disease prevention (Ilich et al., 2014).

In the field of renal health, a comprehensive approach including early detection and timely treatment is crucial to mitigate renal impairment and prevent chronic kidney disease, highlighting the slowness and progression of this pathology (Carrillo-Ucafiay et al., 2022). Preventive strategies must therefore address underlying inflammatory processes, dietary influences and organ-specific vulnerabilities to promote healthy ageing and reduce the burden of age-related diseases.

Geriatrics is now recognised as a science with its own identity, integrating its own disciplines and seeking integration with the basic and clinical sciences, rather than simply being a synthesis of isolated knowledge. Initially, this knowledge was essential for traditional medical practitioners and the survival of chronically ill patients with a poor prognosis. In the context of terminally ill patients, the aim has been to keep the patient in his or her familiar environment, trying to manage crises without necessarily resolving them.In addition, it is crucial to recognise the diseases that most frequently affect the elderly, such as hypertension, which affects 50% of the population over 60 years of age. The main causes of these diseases are cardiovascular diseases, arthropathies (15-30%), rheumatoid arthritis (10%) and osteoarthritis in large joints (Montesino et al., 2022; Âlvarez-Ochoa et al., 2022).

The geriatrician must be able to filter and organise a large amount of disorganised information, skilfully acquiring small doses of technology that will benefit patients. Their work is based on the premise of "healing in particular cases, relieving often and comforting always", following the famous phrase of Francesc de Paula

## 3. Psychological and Social Aspects of Ageing

The ageing of older adults entails a series of psychological changes that involve the acceptance of this process. These changes can generate internal conflicts and the fear of becoming a burden to others, aspects deeply felt by many older people. (Huerta Pozo, 2021).

(Agualongo Chela & Ninabanda Agualongo, 2023) These fears provoke reactions in older people that, although similar to those experienced in previous stages of life, make it difficult for them to adapt to the current environment quickly.

As we age, our personal relationships undergo significant transformations. The ageing process places us in a different socio-affective environment than the one we are used to, affecting our role in society. The psychological changes that accompany ageing, along with the individual characteristics of each person, impact all the social functions in which we participate, including social coping systems that provide support in times of distress or can even be used for economic gain.

Alvear (2024) stresses that man, at birth and death, is a social being. When we reach old age, we experience the phenomenon of ageing, which involves changes in both biology and memory. These changes disaffect the essence of who we are and affect our overall attitude, creating an internal gap and affecting our psycho-emotional sphere.

With ageing, the older person experiences a gradual loss of qualities that define him or her in the eyes of both self and others. This situation can lead to isolation and feelings of maladjustment to the surrounding environment. As we grow in age, our interactions with the environment may become more and more complex. family and social environment tend to diminish, exacerbating these feelings of alienation (Tomala & Rivera, 2023).

### 3.1. Mental and emotional health in old age

Ageing tends to be misinterpreted as physical, emotional and cognitive deterioration. (Iglesias et al.2024) As the years go by, it is true that people experience emotional and cognitive changes, but not all of them are negative.

Studies show that all five emotional dimensions (stress, positive and negative emotions, anxiety and depression) decrease significantly with age. (Camacho Torres & Trejo Bravo, 2023) Both anxiety and depression decrease significantly after the age of 65. This is largely due to cognitive decline associated with ageing, as well as chronic illness and stressful life events. One of the main findings about older adults (over 65 years) is that about half of them may need medical support to improve their quality of life, while the rest learn to tolerate their symptoms and continue with their daily activities. This phenomenon can be accounted for by an analytical approach to coping with the obstacles that arise during old age, as well as by adopting positive or resilient thinking. (Velasco Gaibor, 2022)(Salas et al.2021).

Some salient elements that can contribute to a "successful" old age include: maintaining good health, engaging in rewarding and productive activities, using time creatively, having the ability to adapt to changing and stressful circumstances, coping with life's setbacks in good spirits, having realistic expectations, stimulating cognitive activity through continuing education and interest in current affairs, maintaining an active social life, having a good economic status, or feeling content with what one has.

### 3.2. Adapting to changing roles and circumstances

Becoming a grandparent after the age of 65 often implies the need to modify the patterns of relationships with children, respecting the new role of their partners. This change in family dynamics often coincides with retirement, which allows the grandparent to take on a new role in the relationship with the grandchildren, partially altering the generational dynamics. This role can be very rewarding and compensates, to a certain extent, for leaving the world of work. Therefore, retirement does not necessarily represent a decrease in the number of social roles, but rather a period of adjustment and recombination of previously established roles. For older couples, retirement also means adjusting to longer daily and total cohabitation. This is because, unlike the time spent together during work and weekends, retirement entails a significant increase in the amount of time spent together. In addition, they face the challenge of integrating into the group of older people, which may mean a new social dynamic for them.

In situations where one partner is widowed, it is necessary to adjust to significant changes in their socio-affective situation. Widowhood can complicate the acceptance of this new reality and anticipates challenges in the proper management of illnesses, which are necessary to preserve optimal health. Adapting to widowhood, therefore, involves navigating multiple variables that can make the transition to a new phase of life difficult.

### 3.3. Social support and support networks

Within the framework of stress theory, it is of utmost importance to take into account two essential concepts: the perception of social support and relational socialisation (Cedillo, 2020) (Olivares Ramfrez, 2021). If we start from the premise that a lack of support can generate stress, we can affirm that what really matters is, on the one hand, the relevance of the subjective perception of each individual in a specific situation, in which he or she feels socially supported.

On the other hand, the personal socialisation system is also relevant. From this perspective, human beings have the ability to organise their interpersonal environment in a structured way, depending on the presence or absence of significant others, using variables such as number, quality and stability.

The social organisms that exert influence on the person form a personal network, which can be divided into those significant organisms that have a direct influence on the individual receiving the network, and those whose "role" the subject adheres to (network of relationships). (Reyes Sanchez & Sandoval Bocanegra, 2023).

Support at difficult times and the feeling of being part of a network of rewarding relationships that provide help, appreciation, affection and appropriate information can have significant protective effects on health. Social relationships can provide the individual with a sense of belonging, identity, purpose and orientation based on the roles assumed within the group. Conversely, the absence of meaningful bonds can trigger processes of broad reactivity, making the individual vulnerable to demands for self-attribution of blame. by their situation and the pressures of social norms, which alters self-esteem and generates feelings of isolation (Reyes Sanchez & Sandoval Bocanegra, 2023).

In this context, in the face of threats of loss or when confronted with a norm, the presence of meaningful relationships plays a crucial role through processes of regulation, protection or restriction. This facilitates adaptation to new demands and challenges, demonstrating how meaningful interpersonal connections not only enrich our emotional life, but are also fundamental to our adaptive capacity and psychological well-being.

## 4. Ethical and Legal Aspects in Geriatrics and Gerontology

The elderly population is particularly sensitive and requires ethical considerations that take into account their vulnerability. Although classical bioethical principles are generally applicable, the principles of autonomy, beneficence and non-maleficence are of particular importance for the elderly.

Since the elderly often have a high prevalence of multiple pathologies and in some cases functional limitations, medical care is preferably oriented towards comfort and relief rather than aggressive diagnostic and therapeutic interventions. This helps to avoid institutionalisation and favours the maintenance of the patient's autonomy.

It is crucial that medical interventions respect the patient's wishes and autonomy. It is also vital to ensure that the principles of beneficence and non-maleficence are adhered to, providing comprehensive, quality care that promotes patient autonomy in making decisions about their health.

For the hospitalised elderly, it is important to plan the admission appropriately, avoiding unnecessary urgent actions and the excessive use of complementary tests that will not modify the care plan. Furthermore, technology and medical advances should not displace the importance of a detailed history and physical examination, nor minimise the relevance of maintaining a comprehensive report that reflects the patient's wishes and circumstances.

Informed consent must be obtained for every diagnostic and therapeutic procedure that involves risk, even for minor procedures. This consent should be documented in the medical record, together with the measures taken to support the patient in making related decisions. In the event that the patient signs an informed consent or is admitted to a health care facility, it is essential to clearly identify valid interlocutors in situations where the patient is unable to express his/her wishes. This information should be recorded in the medical record, respecting the applicable legislation, and should include any previous decisions made in specific clinical circumstances, explaining the values and principles accepted by the patient to the patient, his or her family or legal representative, in order to provide the necessary support to make appropriate decisions.

### 4.1. Ethical principles in the care of the elderly

Another important principle in medical ethics is that of 'non-maleficence', i.e. the obligation to do no harm. This principle must be respected both before diagnosing a disease and before proposing a treatment. Linked to this principle is the principle of 'beneficence', i.e. to promote the good of the patient by proposing and applying treatments for the good of the patient and by doing as little harm as possible to the patient.

In addition, the physician is obliged to respect and maintain the confidentiality of all information that reaches him/her through his/her practice, assuming professional secrecy.

This obligation is acquired for a number of reasons. The individual comes to the physician with the confidence that the information he or she provides for treatment will not be disclosed, and the physician cannot perform his or her work effectively without truthful and complete information that can only be obtained by allaying the patient's fears. Therefore, the physician must maintain confidentiality about what the patient tells him or her unless he or she is convinced that failure to disclose the information would result in harm to the individual or to society.

The Code of Medical Ethics states that physicians must respect the dignity of the individual and his or her privacy, both of the elderly and of other persons, avoiding discrimination on the grounds of age. Thus, the only therapeutic alternative for the elderly person should not be the one derived from his or her age, but should take into account clinical judgement and act with equal ethical qualities.

Linked to the dignity of the individual is the principle of autonomy, i.e. the patient has the right to receive the information necessary to make his or her own decisions regarding his or her life and health.

### 4.2. Legislation and rights of the elderly

International humanitarian law is specifically designed to protect older persons. In 1991, the United Nations General Assembly held the World Assembly on Ageing at its headquarters in Vienna: "Towards a Society for All Ages". It reaffirms the human right to a long and healthy life, to legal protection, physical protection and support in old age, considering this objective at national and international level, in the social, economic and humanitarian fields. (Torres et al.2023).

The Charter of Human Rights in Gerontology is a socio-political document that aims to explain, analyse and denounce the complex and variegated phenomenon of ageing in terms of human rights. It also aims to draw attention to the existing reality, its roots and the socio-economic system that underlies it as the immediate cause of other realities and problems that often hide the previous ones.

And in particular, it aims to engage efforts, actions and denunciations with the purpose of fostering social and cultural change among the people involved in different ways: professionals, family members, users and the elderly themselves. (Torres et al.2023).

Legislation related to old age, at international, national and regional level, is nowadays very extensive. This is due to the increase in life expectancy and the growth of the elderly population in Western countries.

Among the fifty countries on the African and intertropical continent, a "Lagos Action Plan" was drawn up, which addresses seven issues related to retired people.

For its part, the Organisation for Economic Co-operation and Development implemented the Statement of Distributive Principles and Recommendations concerning private provision for old age in the twenty most industrialised countries.

Within the European Union, the Maastricht Treaty considers it essential to analyse social expenditure in order to identify situations which exceed the capacities of a state and which, on the other hand, can be financed collectively.

### 4.3. Ethics in geriatric research

Informed consent is of vital importance for the use of data obtained in a research protocol. The geriatric patient should receive extensive information on the study objectives, methodology, possible study treatment alternatives (including standard of care), drug interactions, benefits and potential risks.

Mention should also be made of what makes the procedure difficult to understand, such as the number of medications and tests required. The patient should be given the opportunity to consider this information, either in writing or verbally.

The researcher should ensure that the older adult is confident in the health professional conducting the protocol and not discriminate against those who do not participate, rewarding those who do.Throughout history, there have been situations in which research has compromised the psycho-physical well-being of the geriatric patient who was part of the study. Some authors describe them in a generalised way. For example, Hippocrates mentions the wealthy physicians who conducted unconscionable and unscrupulous research for the sake of prestige and power. In the Nicomachean Ethics, Aristotle mentions that things are judged good or bad in relation to their effects. Galen says that the functionality of the patient should not be compromised for the sake of experimentation. And already in contemporary times, the infamous Nuremberg chain marks the milestone of respect and consideration for the patient who participates in a study.

Today, the participation of older adults in research projects has become crucial in the scientific community, because a significant part of the advances that medicine has achieved in the past has been thanks to the numerous contributions and voluntary participation of people aged 65 years and older.

## 5. Geriatric Assessment Comprehensive

Comprehensive geriatric assessment (CGA) is a fundamental tool in the care of older adults. Despite the importance of IGV, there has been a lack of mobile applications focused on this area, despite its potential to reduce hospitalisations, disability and mortality (Bautista-Mier et al., 2021). IGV is a multidimensional approach that encompasses medical, affective, cognitive, functional, social and spiritual aspects, making it a comprehensive tool for the care of the older adult population (Martfnez et al., 2022). Comprehensive geriatric assessment is of utmost importance in the care and treatment of the elderly population. In contrast to other stages of life, in old age people often face chronic diseases and have less physiological reserve.

These individuals often have difficulty tolerating changes in their internal balance, which often leads to functional disorders secondary to illness and ultimately death. It is essential that medicine for the elderly be able to provide care tailored to these specific characteristics.

### 5.1. Components of geriatric assessment

Comprehensive Geriatric Assessment is a rigorous analysis of the health status of the elderly in order to plan individualised care and treatment.

It is also known as comprehensive geriatric assessment and is a response to the need for the development of assessment programmes for the elderly, focusing on two purposes: to detect and treat acute or chronic disorders in the elderly in order to reduce symptoms and minimise the consequences of the disease; and secondly, to identify and intervene on the specific deficits that contribute to disability and dependency. According to Kirkwood and Melzer, within the assessment of an older adult is the knowledge and consideration of characteristics linked to four distinct but interdependent domains: biological, physiological, pathological and social. The titles of the papers directly emphasise the characteristics analysed in each domain.Each of the components that make up an individual, in isolation, has different characteristics depending on the stage of life in question. However, these characteristics, which are already different in themselves, take on a special value at a stage when there are not as many "resources" available, from a functional, physiological and even pathological point of view, to lead as autonomous a life as possible.

Simultaneous advances in Geriatrics and Gerontology at the end of the 20th century led to a rethinking of this situation. The high prevalence and influence of pathological processes (especially dementia and diseases of the locomotor system) on functional impairment, or the pathological activity underlying the so-called geriatric syndromes (coffee, incontinence and immobilisation), increase the complexity of this already complicated stage of life.

### 5.2. Assessment tools and scales in geriatrics

In the field of geriatrics, the comprehensive geriatric assessment (GGA) plays a crucial role in assessing the health and well-being of older adults. The GGA is a multidimensional tool that considers not only medical aspects but also the emotional, cognitive, functional, social and spiritual dimensions of an individual, making it a key instrument for providing holistic care to older people (Martfnez et al., 2022). This holistic approach is essential for addressing the diverse needs of older adults, especially in the context of terminal illness management, where factors beyond the disease itself can significantly affect outcomes (Beracasa et al., 2021).

While IGV is a valuable tool, its implementation can sometimes be a challenge due to time constraints and lack of standardised methods for geriatric assessments in outpatient settings (Beracasa et al., 2021). In such cases, shorter assessment tools become essential for predicting and efficiently managing treatments in older adults. These shorter tools can provide valuable information on functional performance, cognitive status and social support, which helps in decision-making processes (Beracasa et al., 2021).In the field of geriatric care, the use of mobile applications for comprehensive geriatric assessment is gaining attention for its potential to reduce hospitalisations, institutionalisation, disability and mortality (Bautista-Mier et al., 2021).

While many mobile apps in geriatrics focus on chronic disease management, cognitive stimulation, and physical activity, there is growing recognition of the benefits of incorporating VGI-focused apps into clinical practice. These applications have the potential to revolutionise geriatric care by providing accessible and efficient means to conduct assessments and improve patient outcomes (Bautista-Mier et al., 2021).

Functional assessment is a critical component of geriatric care, especially for identifying limitations and predicting disability in older adults (Ocampo et al., 2017). The implementation of functional assessment tools in clinical practice can help monitor the progression of disabilities and guide care plans for older people, particularly those in institutional settings. By using functional assessment scales, health care providers can better understand the needs of older persons, particularly those in institutional settings. changing needs of older adults and adapt interventions to improve their quality of life

(Ocampo et al., 2017).Depression is a common concern among the elderly population and the Geriatric Depression Scale (GDS) is a widely used tool to assess depressive symptoms in older adults (Almeida and Almeida, 1999). The reliability and validity of the GDS make it a valuable instrument for identifying and managing depression in geriatric patients. Given the high prevalence of depression in the elderly and its impact on general well-being, tools such as the GDS play a crucial role in ensuring comprehensive care for older adults (Almeida and Almeida, 1999).

In the context of pain assessment, numerical rating scales (NRS) are commonly used to assess pain intensity in clinical and research settings (Hidalgo et al., 2021). The NRS allows observers to assign subjective scores to different levels of pain, providing a standardised method for pain assessment. By using tools such as the NRS, healthcare professionals can effectively monitor and manage pain in older adults, thereby improving their quality of life and overall care outcomes (Hidalgo et al., 2021).

In Spanish geriatric services, various assessment tools are used to evaluate the health and functional status of older adults (Ruano et al., 2014). These tools are essential to provide comprehensive care tailored to the specific needs of older adults. By incorporating a variety of assessment instruments, health professionals in Spanish geriatric services can ensure a comprehensive assessment of older patients, leading to more personalised and effective interventions (Ruano et al., 2014).

Nursing assessment in geriatric settings plays a vital role in capturing the holistic needs of older adults, particularly those residing in nursing homes (Sanchez et al., 2007). By using comprehensive nursing assessment tools that encompass various domains, such as physical, mental, social and functional aspects, nurses can develop individualised care plans that address the unique requirements of older residents. These assessment tools serve as a roadmap for providing quality care and promoting the well-being of older adults in institutional settings (Sanchez et al., 2007).

In the context of pressure ulcer risk assessment, the use of standardised scales to assess the risk of developing pressure ulcers is crucial for preventing these debilitating conditions in older adults (Fernandez et al., 2008). These include the Braden scale and the Norton scale. By using validated assessment tools, people at increased risk of pressure ulcers can be identified and specific interventions can be implemented to mitigate these risks. These scales are valuable instruments in geriatric care, as they aid in the early detection and prevention of skin lesions in vulnerable older adults (Fernandez et al., 2008).

The concept of comprehensive geriatric assessment (CGA) is essential in both hospital and primary care settings, as it enables health professionals to provide holistic and high-quality care to older adults (Wanden-Berghe, 2021). Medical staff can gain a holistic understanding of an older patient's health status, functional capacities and social support systems, allowing for personalised interventions that address the individual needs of older people. The holistic approach ensures that older adults receive personalised and effective care that takes into account their unique circumstances and challenges (Wanden-Berghe, 2021). Comprehensive assessment by addressing the patient's different systems (circulatory, respiratory, motor, sensory, psychic) through functional exploration will provide us with the patient's current status and help us to establish the determinant health situations. Some diseases can give rise to geriatric syndromes such as instability, sfncopes, codacides, iatrogenic diseases, functional deterioration and loss of autonomy. These diseases can trigger the most common reasons for consultation in this age group.

Identification of previous illness, diseases in the clinical history that are related to the current condition, location and type should be carried out. An assessment of personal and psychosocial history should also be made. It is important to rule out recent illnesses, infections, malnutrition, fractures, diseases of the nervous system and sequelae of accidents, as well as cases of maltreatment. Unlike the young adult, the older adult has a short-term prognosis and the loss of function rapidly decreases the quality of life. In geriatric analysis, the necessary tools must be used to comprehensively assess the older adult.The multidisciplinary team, consisting of doctors, nurses, physiotherapists, occupational therapists, psychologists and social workers, should seek to obtain maximum information in the assessment and planning of intervention with the older adult. It is essential to use assessment scales appropriate to the context in which they are to be used: whether in out-of-hospital, hospital, residential, home or day-care settings. The time required to complete the scale should be appropriate to the context in which it is applied.

### 5.3. Interpretation of results and care planning

As a resource for identifying changes in the elderly person, professionals have a variety of scales or criteria that bring us closer to the symptomatology.

We can mention the Body Mass Index (BMI), the Snellen visual scale, the Folstein scale, the geriatric depression scale, the MINIMENTAL, among others. All of them should be analysed with a critical attitude, without getting carried away by a single piece of information. It is essential to compile a detailed and accurate medical history, as this guides our interventions towards the needs of the elderly individual. In case of missing personal data, we always look for family members to fill the gap.

We consider as part of normal ageing (within the limits of avoidable pathological loss) declines in body weight, vision or hearing (to some extent); altered mobility, feelings of loneliness or dissatisfaction; decreased sexual desire. Under the term normal ageing, we refer to the functional decline that is to be expected over the years; we consider it generally irreversible and not related to disease. What is important is to find the exact point to identify the pathological situation and to set as a goal the maintenance and recovery of the highest possible level of well-being of the individual.

Normality lies in the total balance and well-being of the human being. As the years go by, the individual experiences a decrease in his or her capacities and many of these pre-pathological signs are perceived as normal in the ageing process (wrinkles in the skin, hair loss, among others).

## 6. Interventions and Treatments at Geriatrics

In the health field, the control of risk factors is crucial, since disease is an irreversible and damaging situation which may nevertheless be amenable to prevention and surveillance, especially in its early stages. The focus is mainly on primary prevention, which aims to prevent the onset of the disease, and secondary prevention, which aims to detect and treat diseases in their early stages. While it is important to prevent disease, it is also crucial to consider that geriatric care focuses largely on alleviating symptoms to improve the patient's well-being. In other words, the aim is to alleviate problems when it would be more effective to adopt preventive measures, since the fewer symptoms that appear, the less treatment will be necessary (Orozco et al., 2024; Pinilla et al., 2020).

(Mufioz Toledo & Ochoa Cueva, 2023) This concept not only focuses on addressing problems from a health perspective, but also on considering the individual's self-perception, social relations and integration in their environment. The attention and care of older adults involves the use of numerous resources and is related to a wide range of problems, strategies and elements to be considered (Castro Silva, 2022).

### 6.1. Pharmacology in old age

The change in distribution volume is unpredictable, as it tends to increase for most drugs, leading to a longer half-life.

The elimination of many drugs is reduced in the elderly, especially through urine. Delayed gastrointestinal function also affects absorption, either due to slower transit (due to decreased smooth muscle tone), mucosal involvement, or drugs such as antacids, which decrease absorption of barbiturates and digoxin.

Altered sensitivity to sympathomimetic and cholinomimetic agonists, changes in brain function, and the effects of stress and chronic illness influence drug behaviour. This variability in drug responses requires regular monitoring of drugs and, where possible, avoidance of their use.

Renal failure and atrophy of numerous organs are of particular relevance. Hepatic and renal changes are relevant, as the liver and kidney are the organs responsible for the metabolism and elimination of most drugs. Generally, the liver will reduce its metabolism of drugs over time, although there are some drugs that do not alter their metabolism. However, there are some exceptions of drugs whose metabolism is affected. Most drugs decrease in renal clearance, which implies a greater pharmacological effect, as their plasma level remains elevated.

### 6.2. Rehabilitation and physiotherapy for the elderly

Physiotherapy acts by improving, from its musculoskeletal field of action, both spastic muscle tone and muscle shortening and hyperlaxity, being recommended in those diseases whose medical treatments do not produce a significant improvement. In the case of degenerative diseases such as Parkinson's disease, physical therapy is not only limited to palliative treatment to be administered in the advanced stages of the disease. However, it is also not possible to completely reduce disabilities in the early stages with new pharmacological actions, so it is necessary to address both movement impairment through appropriate medication and appropriate physiotherapy. These efforts will help to reduce the clear chances of developing motor complications and the risks for both the patient and their relatives. For this reason, it is common to act as if medication can never achieve the desired results in specific movements.

In general, the strategy consists of adapting rehabilitation to the disability that is present and to the medical condition that manifests itself. Thus, apart from a complete geriatric treatment (control of cardiovascular risk factors, detection and treatment of sarcopenia, osteoporosis, etc.), we will add specific physiotherapy for those patients who suffer from it.This will be of great interest to our elderly, especially when there is an inability to perform transfer exercises and active kinesitherapy can hardly be carried out, so active physiotherapy will base its treatment on the inhibition of abnormal reflexes, muscle relaxation, reflex tone inhibition techniques and inhibition of pathological function.

### 6.3. Palliative care and end-of-life care

Palliative care goes beyond the prevention and treatment of pain and other symptoms. It also promotes ethical and humane care for patients and families, as well as assistance with spiritual treatment, all in a dignified and comfortable environment. The aim of palliative care is to control all symptoms generated by a terminal illness, to ensure the best possible quality of life, and to provide support to family members and caregivers. The patient, although aware of the irreversible nature of his or her terminal illness, can and should be involved in all aspects of his or her future plans. The importance of prevention and the comprehensive management of the clinical course of any disease are fundamental reasons to involve all professionals and the medical team in palliative care.

However, the end of life is not always the partial or final result of treatment for a specific disease. Sometimes, death comes as a result of a combination of problems arising from the medical care of partial symptoms or secondary diagnoses, as well as from the limitations of ageing. (Arroyo et al.2022)

The management of this complex situation requires the knowledge and skills of the palliative approach. The physician, who has been the patient's companion throughout his or her life, witnesses the final outcome of a complex physiological evolutionary process, which manifests itself with a final rate of deterioration.

## 7.Research and Advances in Geriatrics and Gerontology

We conclude this section by highlighting, in general terms, some of the areas of knowledge in which the most significant advances in Geriatrics and Gerontology have been made in the last two decades.

Research in this field has led to a better understanding and analysis of the specific health problems of the elderly population, while identifying and developing more appropriate interventions and determining their impact on the health and quality of life of the elderly patient. Among the areas that have been identified as the most advanced are: all aspects related to the normal ageing process and chronic diseases affecting the elderly.

Project development: There are many organisations carrying out research support programmes in the fields of Geriatrics and Gerontology. In Europe, IAGG-Europe has established a network to exchange ideas and encourage the creation of joint proposals, allowing them to circulate among its members. While respecting the particularities of each country, proposals at national level as well as those specifically addressed to international organisations and their various programmes are equally relevant.

Implementation of the research: Project implementation involves the need for patient search, data collection, field work, laboratory work, sample analysis. In addition to time-consuming administrative procedures often involved, there are multiple entities equipped with infrastructures and methods to facilitate the practical part of the research.

### 7.1. Basic and clinical research in gerontology

Basic and clinical research in gerontology is essential to better understand the processes of ageing and to develop more effective treatments for older adults. In addition, it provides an in-depth understanding of age-related diseases and helps to find ways to prevent and treat them more efficiently.

Basic research provides the essential foundation on the primordial nature of certain processes that condition the object of knowledge itself.

On the other hand, clinical research employs methods and techniques to unravel answers to specific questions related to the disease. The lack of clinical research has a direct impact on the insufficient level of knowledge of the preventive and therapeutic aspects of the disease in general in older people. Also, the lack of knowledge about clinical manifestations, pathogenesis and pathophysiology of diseases with a high incidence in the elderly or the use and effects of drug administration on the organism of the elderly constitute a major obstacle to the development of the discipline.

Most research in the basic sciences lacks a clinical orientation, since its aim is to study fundamental and universal processes that allow us to know the general laws of nature, which constitutes so-called pure science. On the other hand, the ultimate purpose or applied level of clinical research is achieved only in the acquisition of concrete information that can be useful in daily clinical practice or treatment planning.

It is therefore clear that the approach to the needs of the elderly and thus the quality of daily clinical information is directly dependent on the development of research.

### 7.2. Innovative technologies and approaches in elderly care

In the field of geriatrics and gerontology, multiple technologies and innovative approaches have been developed in order to improve the care of older adults. One such development is the use of remote monitoring devices, which allow healthcare professionals to constantly track patients' vital parameters from the comfort of their homes. These devices include activity sensors, blood pressure monitors and glucose monitors. In addition, mobile applications and digital platforms have been developed to foster communication between patients and their doctors, streamlining care and reducing the need for travel (Acufia Valderrama, 2022)(Vega Baudrit et al., 2024)(Mufioz Zuta).

Another innovative approach lies in the use of virtual reality and augmented reality to improve rehabilitation and physiotherapy for the elderly. These technologies enable the recreation of virtual environments that facilitate the performance of exercises and physical activities, stimulating mobility and functionality. In short, innovative technologies and approaches in the care of older adults are transforming the way their care is addressed and improving their quality of life (Collazo et al., 2020) (Vega Baudrit et al., 2024).

### 7.3. Future perspectives and challenges

Geriatrics and gerontology face a number of challenges and have promising prospects for the future. One of the main challenges is the ageing population and the increasing demand for specialised medical care for the elderly.

This requires the development of education and training programmes in geriatrics and gerontology to ensure that health professionals are prepared to address the needs of this population.

In addition, there is a need to improve research in this area in order to develop innovative approaches and effective treatments for the care of the elderly.

Future perspectives include the use of advanced healthcare technology, such as telemedicine and artificial intelligence, to offer more accessible and personalised services to the elderly. Greater emphasis is also expected on health promotion and disease prevention in old age, through public policy and education programmes.

In summary, geriatrics and gerontology face major challenges but also have great potential to improve the quality of life of the elderly in the future.

## REFERENCES


• Acufia Valderrama, J. A. (2022). Disefio de un sistema de monitoreo de patients with ambulatory diseases, in support of a general care health facility, category II 1, of the ... utp.edu.pe

• Agualongo Chela, L. G. & Ninabanda Agualongo, S. M. (2023). Pathology-related emotional changes; COVID 19 in older adults.

Centro de Salud Promejoras San Camilo precinct January-April 2023.ueb.edu.ec

• Âlvarez-Ochoa, R., Torres-Criollo, L. M., Ortega, J. P. G., Coronel, D. C. I., Cayamcela, D. M. B., Pelaez, V. D. R. L., & Salinas, A. S. S. (2022). Risk factors for hypertension in adults. A critical review. Revista Latinoamericana de Hipertensi6n, 17(2). ucv.ve

• Alvear, M. E. C. (2024). Envejecimiento humano: un analisis integral desde la perspectiva de la medicina interna. RECIAMUC. reciamuc.com

• Amarya, S., Singh, K., & Sabharwal, M. (2018). Ageing process and physiological changes... https://doi.org/10.5772/intechopen.76249

• Arias, C., Soliverez, C., & Bozzi, N. (2020). El envejecimiento poblacionalen América Latina: Aportes para el delineamiento de polfticas publicas. Revista Euro latinoamericana de Analisis Social y Polftico (RELASP), 1(2), 11-23. unr.edu.ar

• Arroyo, L. I., Ortega-Lenis, D., Ardila, L., Leal, F., Morales, O., Calvache, J. A., & De Vries, E. (2022). Physician perceptions of end-of-life care in oncology patients. Revista Gerencia y Polfticas de Salud, 21, 1-21. redalyc.org.

• Athar, A., Dhaduk, K., & Aronow, W. (2019). Pericardial diseases in elderly patients... https://doi.org/10.5772/intechopen.89473

• Ballesteros, F. Z. (2023). KNEE OSTEOARTHRITIS, OSTEOMUSCULAR HEALTH AND

PHYSICAL ACTIVITY IN THE ELDERLY. EmasF, Revista Digital de Educaci6n Ffsica, 15(85). webcindario.com

• BALTASAR, M. C., MENDOZA, M. D., & LOPEZ-REY, C. A. (). LITERATURE REVIEW: DYSPHAGIA IN THE OLDER ADULT. publicacionescientificas.es. publicacionescientificas.es

• Bautista-Mier, H., Rodrfguez-Gutiérrez, A., Torres-Espinosa, C., & L6pez- Ramfrez, J. (2021). Use and perception of a mobile application for comprehensive geriatric assessment by health care personnel. Medunab, 24(2), 169-182. https://doi.org/10.29375/01237047.4041

• Beracasa, L., Bar6n, C., & Sanchez, J. (2021). Cancer treatment-related toxicity in older adults. review of the literature. Universitas Médica, 62(1). https://doi.org/10.11144/javeriana.umed62- 1.toxi

• Bertolotti, L. (2022). Cognitive functioning in ageing: psychopedagogical intervention. ufasta.edu.ar

• Bora, A., Koç, M., Durmus, K., & Altunta□, E. (2021). Evaluating the frequency of

anatomical variations of the sinonasal region in pediatric and adult age.
groups according to gender: computed tomography findings of 1532 cases.
The Egyptian Journal of Otolaryngology, 37(1). https://doi.org/10.1186/s43163-021-00122-9

• Burgos, L. E. M., Âlvarez, R. E. Z., Bermudez, L. S. M., & Cedefio, C. I. M. (2023). Prevention of advanced chronic diseases and public health. RECIAMUC, 7(2), 55-64. reciamuc.com.

• Camacho Torres, L. V. & Trejo Bravo, F. V. (2023). La ansiedad en el proceso de envejecimiento de los/as adultos/as mayores del Centro De Salud Tipo C "Basti6n Popular" de la ciudad de Guayaquil en el periodo de ... ups.edu.ec

• Castro Silva, J. Y. (2022). Propuesta de modelo de atenci6n con enfoque de desarrollo humano sostenible para mejorar la calidad de vida de adultos mayores. Chachapoyas. untrm.edu.pe

• Cedillo, G. J. (2020). Social work in health: theory and innovative praxis. Margen: journal of social work and social sciences. academia.edu

• CISNEROS, L. O. (2021). Telomerase activity and cell cycle regulation during the transition from the neurogenesis phase to the gliogenesis phase in the spinal cord. unam.mx

• Collazo, C., Santos, J. G., Bernal, J. G., & Cubo, E. (2020). Status on the status of the use and potential utilities of new technologies for measuring physical activity. Systematic review of the literature. Attention
Practical Primary. sciencedirect.com

• Criollo, W. (2019). Assessment of functional capacity and activities of daily living in institutionalized older adults. Scientific Movement,
13(2). https://doi.org/10.33881/2011-7191.mct.13201

• Duque-Fernandez, L. M., Ornelas-Contreras, M., & Benavides-Pando, E. V. (2020). Physical activity and its relationship to aging and functional capacity: a review of the research literature. Psicologfa y Salud, 30(1), 45-57. uv.mx

• Furuya, J., Tamada, Y., Sato, T., Hara, A., Nomura, T., Kobayashi, T., - & Kondo, H. (2015). Wearing complete dentures is associated with changes in the three-dimensional shape of the oropharynx in edentulous older people that affect swallowing. Gerodontology, 33(4), 513-521. https://doi.org/10.1111/ger.12197

• Gallegos, W., Toia, A., & Rivera, R. (2021). Analisis psicométrico de la escala de de depresi6n geriatrica de yesavage en adultos mayores de la macroregi6n sur del peru. Revista Enfermeria Herediana, 12, 11-19. https://doi.org/10.20453/renh.v12i0.3960

• Garcfa Montes de Oca, A. L. & in Estomatologfa, E. P. G. (). THE DETERIORATION OF MASTICATORY FUNCTION AND THE INFLUENCE OF NUTRITION ON THE OLDER ADULT. THE IMPAIRMENT OF MASTICATION ... cisalud-.
ucmh.sld.cu. sld.cu

• Gondim, E., Moreira, M., Lima, A., Aquino, P., & Nascimento, S. (2022). Women know about perineal trauma risk but do not know how to prevent it: knowledge, attitude, and practice. International Journal of Gynecology & Obstetrics, 161(2), 470-477.

https://doi.org/10.1002/ijgo.14526
• Gonzalez-Montalvo, J. I., Ramfrez-Martfn, R., Colino, R. M., Alarc6n, T., Tarazona-Santabalbina, F. J., Martfnez-Velilla, N., ... & Martfn-Sanchez, F. J. (2020). Transversal geriatrics. A healthcare challenge for the 21st century. Revista Espafiola de Geriatrfa y Gerontologfa, 55(2), 84-97. [HTML].
• Grande Aranda, J. I. (2024). The vulnerable: interdisciplinary studies on vulnerability. [HTML].
• Huerta Pozo, K. (2021). Influencia de cambios sociales en los sentimientos del proceso de envejecimiento "Centro Integral del Adulto Mayor"- Municipalidad Provincial de Huanuco 2019. 200.37.135.58
• Iglesias, S. R., Preciado, M. C. R., & Carrasco, L. Y. V. (2024). Impacto del Programa Social Pensi6n 65 en la satisfacci6n de necesidades de adultos mayores peruanos. Revista InveCom/ISSN en lfnea: 2739-0063, 4(2), 1-10. revistainvecom.org.
• Jernigan, T., Archibald, S., Berhow, M., Sowell, E., Foster, D., & Hesselink, J. (1991). Cerebral structure on mri, part i: localization of age-related changes. Biological Psychiatry, 29(1), 55-67. https://doi.org/10.1016/0006- 3223(91)90210-d
• Juna, H. and Paez, M. (2023). Creation and validation of the nursing health assessment format for geriatric patients. Brazilian Journal of Health Review, 6(1), 2815-2827. https://doi.org/10.34119/bjhrv6n1-221
• Kanasi, E., Ayilavarapu, S., & Jones, J. (2016). The aging population: demographics and the biology of aging. Periodontology 2000, 72(1), 13-18. https://doi.org/10.1111/prd.12126
• LA, V. FINAL EPILOGUE. wordpress.com
• Landazabal, O. S. & Barboza, F. Y. A. (2020). Derechos humanos del adulto mayor en el ambito familiar colombiano en el marco del envejecimiento demografico. Jurfdicas CUC. unirioja.es
• Lemaître, H., Goldman, A., Sambataro, F., Verchinski, B., Meyer-Lindenberg, A., Weinberger, D., - & Mattay, V. (2012). Normal age-related brain morphometric changes: nonuniformity across cortical thickness, surface area and gray matter volume? Neurobiology of Aging, 33(3), 617.e1-617.e9. https://doi.org/10.1016/j.neurobiolaging.2010.07.013
• Malan Valente, A. B. (2024). Humanizaci6n en el cuidado del adulto mayor en el area de hospitalizaci6n del Hospital Basico Guamote. udla.edu.ec
• Martfnez, D., Martfnez, A., Sanchez, M., & Ramos, S. (2022). Importancia de la valoraci6n geriatrica integral a prop6sito de un caso. Investigaci6n Y Desarrollo, 10(1), 56-60. https://doi.org/10.31243/id.v10.2016.182
• Mazzini, M. B. B., Salazar, M. F. B., Sanchez, J. P. E., & Amaya, J. E. R. (2023). Comprehensive geriatric assessment for older adults. Polo del Conocimiento: Revista cientffico-profesional, 8(6), 1453-1473. unirioja.es
• Montesino, D. C., Reguera, I. P., Fernandez, O. R., Relova, M. R., & Valladares, W. C. (2022). Clinical and epidemiological characterization of disability in the older adult population. Interdisciplinary Rehabilitation/Rehabilitacion Interdisciplinaria, 2, 15-15. saludcyt.ar

• Mufioz Toledo, M. B. & Ochoa Cueva, I. S. (2023). Calidad de vida del adulto mayor en una comunidad segun Betty Neuman. ucacue.edu.ec
• Mufioz Zuta, J. L. (). Design of an intelligent monitoring system intradomiciliario y remoto para el cuidado de la población adultaci6n mayor. tesis.pucp.edu.pe. pucp.edu.pe
• Ney, D., Weiss, J., Kind, A., & Robbins, J. (2009). Senescent swallowing: impact, strategies, and interventions. Nutrition in Clinical Practice, 24(3), 395-413. https://doi.org/10.1177/0884533609332005
• Nigam, Y., Knight, J., Bhattacharya, S., & Bayer, A. (2012). Physiological changes associated with aging and immobility. Journal of Aging Research, 2012, 1-2. https://doi.org/10.1155/2012/468469
• Nufiez, D. (2017). Comprehensive geriatric assessment in older adults with cancer. Revista Clfnica Escuela De Medicina Ucr-HSJD, 7(3). https://doi.org/10.15517/rc_ucr-hsjd.v7i3.30018
• Ocampo, D., Mufioz, I., & G6mez, F. (2017). Prediction of performance measures in institutionalized wheelchair-bound elderly. Revista Colombiana De Rehabilitaci6n, 12(1), 6. https://doi.org/10.30788/revcolreh.v12.n1.2013.45
• Olivares Ramfrez, F. (2021). Perception of family functionality and social support in patients with disability due to Covid 19 in the HGZ1 Delegation Aguascalientes. uaa.mx
• Orozco, J. C., Diaz, J. R. D. L. O., & Brenes, A. G. M. (2024). Aproximaci6n a la Intervenci6n de la Demencia desde los Cuidados Paliativos. Ciencia Latina: Revista Multidisciplinar, 8(1), 690-708. unirioja.es
• Parrales, G. L. P. & Molina, S. A. A. (2020). The family in the care of older adults. utm.edu.ec
• Pinilla, J. M. G., Dfez-Villanueva, P., Freire, R. B., Formiga, F., Marcos, M. C., Bonanad, C., ... & Martfnez-Sellés, M. (2020). Consensus document and recommendations on palliative care in heart failure from the Heart Failure and Geriatric Cardiology Sections of the Spanish Society of Cardiology. Revista espafiola de cardiologfa, 73(1), 69-77. [HTML]
• Pifia Moran, M., Olivo Viana, M. G., Martfnez Matamala, C., Poblete Troncoso, M., & Guerra Guerrero, V. (2022). Ageing, quality of life and health. Challenges to the social roles of older people. Rumbos TS, 17(28), 7-27. scielo.cl
• Ramfrez, G. E. R. (2023). La Biologfa Molecular del envejecimiento. Ciencia Latina Revista Cientffica Multidisciplinar. ciencialatina.org
• Reyes Sanchez, L. P. & Sandoval Bocanegra, V. A. (2023). Stress, depression and social support in older adults. ucv.edu.pe
• Reyna, R., Contreras, M., & Vega, H. (2021). Use of the SF-36 Health Questionnaire in older adults. Systematic review. Anxiety and stress. researchgate.net
• Salas Zapata, C., Aguilar G6mez, M., Giraldo Sanchez, T. E., Mufioz Rua, M. C., Torres Bland6n, A., Uribe Castafio, A., & Uribe Quintero, A. (2021). Major depression in the general population of Envigado (Colombia): prevalence and associated factors. CES Psicologfa, 14(3), 117-133. scielo.org.co
• Scilimati, N., Beccati, F., Dall'Aglio, C., Meo, A., & Pepe, M. (2022). Age and sex

correlate with bony changes and anatomic variations of the lumbosacroiliac region of the vertebral column in a mixed population of horses. Journal of the American Veterinary Medical Association, 1-8. https://doi.org/10.2460/javma.22.07.0293. https://doi.org/10.2460/javma.22.07.0293

• Tomala, F. & Rivera, S. N. Y. (2023). Family abandonment and emotional state of older adults in the Parafso neighbourhood of Salinas canton.... 593 Digital Publisher CEIT. unirioja.es

• Torres, A., Pérez-Galavfs, A., Ron, M., & Mendoza, N. (2023). Psychosocial Workplace Factors and Stress in Medical Care Personnel. Interdisciplinary Rehabilitation/Rehabilitacion Interdisciplinaria, 3, 42-42. healthcyt.co.uk

• Vega Baudrit, J., Corrales, R., Castillo Henrfquez, L., & Camacho, M. (2024). Telemedicine and the Internet of Medical Things (IoMT): Overcoming challenges and visualising opportunities to improve the quality of life and accessibility in the health sector. ulead.ac.cr

• Velasco Gaibor, C. E. (2022). Abandonment of the family and its influence on the emotional state of a 65-year-old woman hospitalised in the Atalaya Gerontol6gic Residential Centre in Chillanes canton.... 190.15.129.146

• Wanden-Berghe, C. (2021). Comprehensive geriatric assessment. Hospital at Home, 5(2), 115. https://doi.org/10.22585/hospdomic.v5i2.136

• Yungplut, F. (2024). Diagnostic and therapeutic strategies used in non-institutionalised patients over 70 years of age based on functional loss of physical abilities.. ufasta.edu.ar

• Zarebski, G. (2021). The World Health Organization (WHO): From Healthy Ageing to Old Age as a Disease. Challenges for Gerontology. IGERMED Journal. inicien.com

• Zubiria, L. M. A. (2024). Desaffos y perspectivas de la polftica publica del envejecimiento en Colombia. Revista Venezolana de Gerencia: RVG. unirioja.es

# CHAPTER 2
# B-LEARNING

In recent decades, a number of different approaches have been employed to use ICT (information and communication technologies) to support teaching and learning in higher education.

The trend is towards the integration of mobile technology (tablets, smartphones, portable servers) with flexible pedagogical approaches such as integrated classrooms, constructive makerspaces and gamification (Becker et al. 2018; Johnson et al. 2014).

Virtual education trends have experienced exponential development since the COVID 19 pandemic, the latest Horizon Report (Alexander et al. 2019) described a situational analysis in favour of trends such as mobile learning and analytics technologies; and in the near future, artificial intelligence (AI) is expected to play more important roles in education. This situation is already occurring today, and it is anticipated that developments in the near future will focus on blockchain and virtual assistants for educational learning support.

It is in this context that E leraning (e-learning) emerged which allows synchronous and asynchronous sessions and the repetition of content for better visual fixation (Tan and Erdogan, 2004; Yal n, 2000). However, asynchronous E-learning suffers from some limitations widely described in the literature; such as students' perceived sense of isolation and lack of motivation (Dogan, Duman & Seferoglu, 2011); as well as poor communication and social interaction with the teacher and between peers.

Thus, B-learning emerged as a learning process that integrates aspects of face-to-face and online learning through the use of e-learning technologies applied to traditional learning environments.

Its benefits were quickly realised, such as an effective speed of individual learning and the creation of more flexible learning environments.

B leraning can be defined as an educational approach that combines traditional face-to-face instruction with online learning activities (Amponsah, 2020). It is characterised by the integration of technology into the learning process, allowing for a flexible and personalised learning experience (Valtonen et al., 2020).

B learning provides pedagogical support through a variety of methods, including lectures, formative quizzes, automated assessment, self- and peer-assessment, and online forums for peer support and discussion (Glance et al., 2013). This combination of instructional strategies promotes active learning, participation and collaboration among students (Boston- Hill et al., 2021).

ELEMENTOS DEL APRENDIZAJE COMBINADO
Componente Presencial o cara a cara
Salones de clase virtuales
Comunicación vía correo electrónico
Instrucción interactiva basada en la Web
Foros de discusión electrónica
Contenido para aprendizaje autónomo
Conferencias vía computador
Video conferencia-Audio conferencia

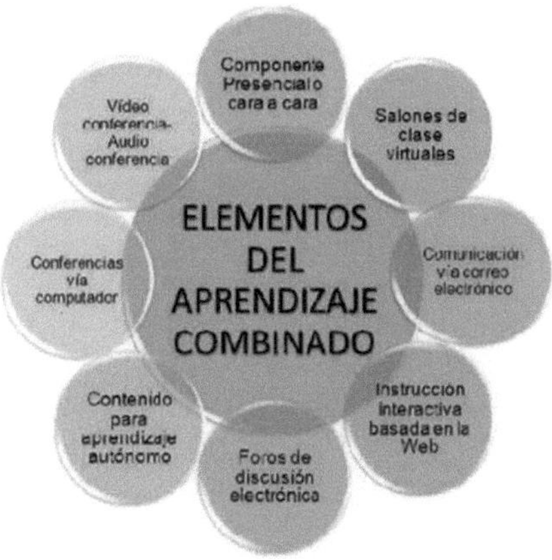

Features

https://linnealab.wordpress.com

The main characteristics of blended learning are (Dangwal, K. L. (2017)...:

• Students have the opportunity of both modalities: blended learning allows in its traditional component to get personal interaction with the teacher and their peers and to complement their learning with ICT support.

• This depends largely on the nature of the content and the objectives, which are designed by the teachers, who choose the appropriate method.

• For a correct application, teachers must be familiar with both methodologies. A fundamental characteristic is the dynamism and technical training to migrate between the traditional classroom format and the online format.

the ICT-supported format. This is closely related to the availability of IT infrastructure and resources.

• Students develop competencies in the use of new technologies and gain the ability to exploit the available technologies to their fullest advantage.

• It allows the integral development of the personality. In areas such as cognitive, physical and emotional. Traditional classroom teaching is useful at the memory level and the cognitive comprehension level and is complemented by online activities. Self-managed experiences help at the reflective level of learning.

• Students gain broad exposure and new perspectives on the subject content, their content knowledge is enriched, they can develop new dimensions of practice and meaningful learning.

• The role of the teacher in blended learning is diversified beyond the traditional one; he/she becomes a motivator, facilitator, organiser and developer of content through ICT.

They have the opportunity to develop their professional growth.

• The student constructs knowledge rather than simply repeating it; A model of constructivism is developed where students become self-managing and self-effective in their academic and personal development.

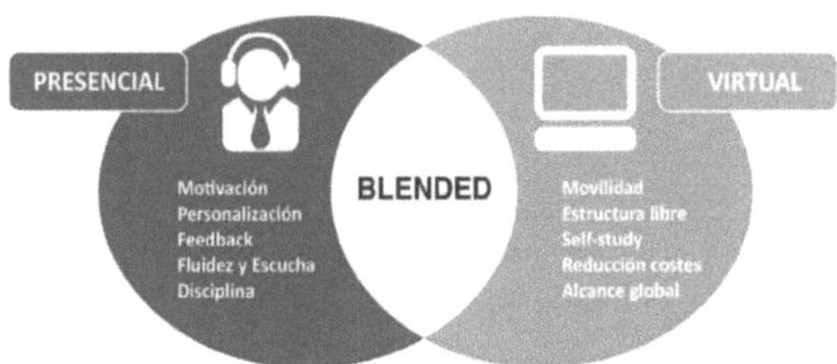


Benefits

One of the benefits of B learning in higher education is its ability to cater for different learning styles and preferences (Amponsah, 2020). By incorporating both online and face-to-face components, B learning allows students to interact with course materials in a way that is tailored to their individual learning styles (Amponsah, 2020). their individual needs. This flexibility promotes self-directed learning and allows students to take ownership of their education (Amponsah, 2020). In addition, B-learning provides opportunities for students to develop digital literacy skills, which are essential in today's technology-driven society (Vlachopoulos & Makri, 2017).

The study by Cobanoglu, A. et al (2014) demonstrated benefits in 2 main areas: Academic performance, although not significantly in relation to face-to-face activity (depending on the pedagogical designs implemented and motivational factors); Perception of cognitive flexibility, students developed metacognitive activities and discovered different points of view when interacting with peers.

Limitations

However, B-learning also has its limitations. One limitation is the potential for unequal access to technology and internet connectivity, which can create disparities in learning opportunities (Meskhi et al., 2019). Another constraint is the need for effective time management and self-regulation skills, as B-learning requires learners to take responsibility for their own learning and stay motivated (Valtonen et al., 2020). In addition, the design and implementation of B-learning courses require careful planning and consideration of instructional strategies to ensure that online and face-to-face components are seamlessly integrated (Herrington and Herrington, 2006).

Perspectives

Despite these limitations, B-learning has promising prospects in higher education. It offers the potential to improve the quality of education by combining the best aspects of traditional instruction with the advantages of online learning (Valtonen et al., 2020). B-learning can also facilitate collaboration and communication among students and between students and instructors, fostering a sense of community and engagement (Boston-Hill et al., 2021). In addition, B-learning can provide opportunities for lifelong learning and professional development, as it allows individuals to access educational resources and participate in courses from anywhere and at any time (Amponsah, 2020).

**Conclusion**

In conclusion, B-learning in higher education is a pedagogical approach that combines face-to-face instruction with online learning activities. It provides pedagogical support through a variety of methods and promotes active learning and collaboration. B learning offers benefits such as flexibility, personalised learning and the development of digital literacy skills. However, it also has limitations related to access to technology and the need for effective time management. Despite these limitations, B-learning has promising prospects in higher education, including improving the quality of education, fostering community and engagement, and facilitating lifelong learning and professional development.

## REFERENCES

• Amponsah, S. (2020). Exploring the dominant learning styles of adult learners in higher education. International Review of Education, 66(4), 531-550. https://doi.org/10.1007/s11159-020-09845-y

• Becker, S., Brown, M., Dahlstrom, E., Davis, A., DePaul, K., Diaz, V., et al. (2018). NMC Horizon report: 2018 higher (education ed.). Louisville, CO: EDUCAUSE.

• Boston-Hill, K., Stelljes, D., Boersma, J., & Boersma, J. (2021). Debate for civic learning: a model for renewing higher education's civic mission. Journal of the Scholarship of Teaching and Learning, 21(4). https://doi.org/10.14434/josotl.v21i4.32845

• Cobanoglu, A., & Yurdakul, B. (2014). The Effect of Blended Learning on Students' Achievement, Perceived Cognitive Flexibility Levels and Self- Regulated Learning Skills*. Journal of Education and Practice, 5, 176-196.

• Dangwal, K. L. (2017). Blended learning: An innovative approach. Universal Journal of Educational Research, 5(1), 129-136.

• Glance, D., Forsey, M., & Riley, M. (2013). The pedagogical foundations of massive open online courses. First Monday. https://doi.org/10.5210/fm.v18i5.4350

• Herrington, A. and Herrington, J. (2006). What is an authentic learning environment?., 1-14. https://doi.org/10.4018/978-1-59140-594-8.ch001

• Meskhi, B., Ponomareva, S., & Ugnich, E. (2019). E-learning in higher inclusive education: needs, opportunities and limitations. International Journal of Educational Management, 33(3), 424-437.https://doi.org/10.1108/ijem-09-2018-0282

• Valtonen, T., Leppanen, U., Hyypia, M., Kokko, A., Manninen, J., Vartiainen, H.,& Hirsto, L. (2020). Learning environments preferred by university students: a shift toward informal and flexible learning environments. LearningEnvironments Research, 24(3), 371-388. https://doi.org/10.1007/s10984-020-09339-6

• Vlachopoulos, D. and Makri, A. (2017). The effect of games and simulations on higher education: a systematic literature review. International Journal of Educational Technology in Higher Education, 14(1). https://doi.org/10.1186/s41239-017-0062-1

# CHAPTER 3
# TEACHING GERIATRIC SYNDROMES TO RESIDENT PHYSICIANS THROUGH B-LEARNING

## Introduction

In the field of geriatric medicine, adequate training in the management of geriatric syndromes is crucial due to the growing number of older adults and the complex health needs associated with this population. Geriatric syndromes, such as immobility, drowsiness, urinary incontinence, cognitive impairment, sarcopenia and frailty, present unique challenges that require a specialised and comprehensive approach. This book is designed to equip resident physicians with the knowledge and skills necessary to diagnose, treat and manage these syndromes effectively, using the B-learning method.

B-learning or blended learning combines elements of traditional face-to-face learning and e-learning techniques to create a richer and more flexible educational experience. This approach facilitates deeper understanding and self-directed learning, allowing residents to interact with both digital content and hands-on experience. In this context, B-learning is particularly well suited to the teaching of geriatric syndromes, as it allows for the incorporation of multiple educational resources, such as simulations, videoconferencing, discussion forums and hands-on activities. The teaching of geriatric syndromes to medical residents is a fundamental aspect of their education and training. Geriatric syndromes, which occur frequently in the geriatric population, are clinical conditions that affect the health and well-being of older adults. The aim of this course is to provide resident physicians with the knowledge necessary to recognise, diagnose and appropriately treat the different geriatric syndromes. Through the b-learning approach, which combines face-to-face education with e-learning, the course is designed to provide the necessary knowledge to recognise, diagnose and appropriately treat the different geriatric syndromes. The aim is to provide comprehensive and up-to-date training that will enable resident doctors to acquire the competencies necessary for the optimal care of geriatric patients. This section will introduce the topic, highlighting the importance of teaching geriatric syndromes and their relationship to b-learning.

This chapter will address each specific geriatric syndrome, and is designed to serve as a comprehensive guide to effective teaching and learning. By the end of each chapter, residents will not only have acquired theoretical knowledge, but will also have developed practical skills through interactive exercises and case studies designed to replicate real-world challenges. In addition, the integration of information technologies and e-learning platforms ensures that resident physicians can continue their training in a continuous and adaptive manner, responding to the changing demands of the geriatric field. This chapter aims not only to educate but also to inspire future geriatricians to adopt a holistic and empathetic approach to the care of the elderly, thus improving both their quality of life and their dignity. With an emphasis on educational innovation and practical application, we aim to set a new standard in geriatric medical training.

1. Definition of Geriatric Syndromes

Geriatric syndromes refer to a set of multifactorial and common diseases in the geriatric population that are characterised by the presence of specific clinical signs and symptoms. These are heterogeneous conditions that include immobility, coffees, cognitive impairment, sarcopenia and frailty.These syndromes occur as a result of the interaction of multiple factors and their diagnosis is based on the identification of the corresponding clinical criteria.It is important to emphasise that these syndromes should not be considered as isolated diseases, but rather as multiple and interrelated clinical manifestations. Their approach and treatment require a multidisciplinary approach involving different medical specialties in order to improve the quality of life of geriatric patients and prevent further complications.In this regard, collaboration between geriatricians, physiotherapists, nutritionists, psychologists and social workers is crucial to establish comprehensive care plans that effectively address each syndrome individually and together. It is essential to bear in mind that many of these geriatric syndromes increase the risk of disability, hospitalisation and mortality in older people, so their early detection and appropriate management are essential aspects of geriatric health care. Therefore, it is crucial to promote awareness and training in the management of these syndromes in both clinical and community settings in order to ensure comprehensive and quality care for the geriatric population. (Pefia et al.2020)(Corzo Camacho).

2. Classification of Geriatric Syndromes

The classification of geriatric syndromes allows for the organisation and categorisation of the different types of medical conditions affecting older people. Among the most common geriatric syndromes are: immobility syndrome, characterised by loss of movement and functional ability; caudaemia syndrome, which refers to recurrent caudaemia and its consequences in older adults; cognitive impairment syndrome, which involves the progressive loss of mental abilities; sarcopenia, which is the loss of muscle mass and strength in the elderly; and frailty syndrome, which is characterised by decreased endurance and physical vulnerability. Each of these syndromes has its own specific definition, epidemiology, diagnosis, assessment tools and specific approach and treatment, which is essential for providing comprehensive and effective geriatric care.

a. Immobility Syndrome

• Definition and Clinical Relevance

Immobility in the elderly population is defined as the partial or total loss of the ability to move and perform physical activities independently. This geriatric syndrome is of particular clinical interest because of its profound implications for the quality of life and general health of the elderly. Immobility significantly increases the risk of complications such as pressure ulcers, venous thrombosis, respiratory infections and psychosocial deterioration, among others. It is characterised by the absence of physical activity or restriction of movement due to various underlying conditions, such as chronic illness, disability or cognitive impairment. According to epidemiology, this syndrome affects a high percentage of older people, especially in long-term care settings. The diagnosis of immobility syndrome is based on clinical assessment of mobility, muscle strength and functional capacity. For this purpose, assessment tools such as mobility assessment scales and specific physical tests are used. The approach and treatment of immobility syndrome includes non-pharmacological interventions such as physiotherapy, adapted physical exercise and occupational therapy, which aim to improve mobility and prevent complications associated with immobility. In addition, pharmacological strategies for symptom management and pain control may be considered.

It is essential that medical residents acquire solid knowledge about this syndrome, since its early detection and adequate treatment are crucial to improve the quality of life and prevent disability in the geriatric population (Tamayo Pérez, 2023) (Suarez Tomala, 2022).

• Risk Factors and Consequences

Risk factors for immobility include advanced age, chronic diseases such as arthritis and Parkinson's disease, accidents, surgical operations and post-stroke states. Early identification of these factors in geriatric patients is crucial for effective prevention and management. The consequences of immobility not only affect the physical health of the elderly, but also their emotional and social well-being, often leading to a cycle of deterioration that can be difficult to reverse.

• Epidemiology

Immobility syndrome is a common health problem in the geriatric population. According to epidemiological studies, it is estimated that about 60% of institutionalised older adults and 30% of community-dwelling older adults have immobility syndrome. The prevalence of immobility increases with age, being more common in people over 80 years of age. This condition is associated with an increased risk of medical complications and reduced quality of life. The epidemiology of immobility syndrome underlines the importance of its recognition and appropriate management in the training of resident doctors, with the aim of to improve the care of geriatric patients (Tamayo Pérez, 2023)(MUNOZ).

• Diagnosis

The diagnosis of immobility is based on functional assessment of the patient, using tools such as the Timed Up and Go Mobility Scale (TUG) and the Stand and Walk Test. In addition, specific assessment instruments such as the Tinetti Test can be used to assess functionality and risk of falls. In addition, a comprehensive assessment including cognitive, emotional and social aspects is essential for a more complete approach. The diagnosis of Immobility Syndrome is based on clinical assessment and the detection of signs and symptoms characteristic of lack of mobility in the elderly. The patient's medical history should be considered, as well as a complete physical assessment including tests of muscle strength, balance and the ability to perform basic activities of daily living. Early and accurate diagnosis of Immobility Syndrome is essential in order to implement an appropriate approach and treatment, with the aim of improving quality of life and preventing complications in geriatric patients.

• Valuation Instruments

Some of the most commonly used instruments are the Tinetti scale to assess balance and gait, the Timed Up and Go test to measure mobility, and the Mini-Mental State Examination (MMSE) to assess cognitive function. These tools are of great use to the resident physician, as they allow him/her to obtain accurate and objective information for the diagnosis and follow-up of geriatric syndromes, thus facilitating the implementation of an appropriate approach and effective treatment.

• Approach and treatment

The management of immobility requires a multidisciplinary approach, including physiotherapy to improve strength and balance, nutritional intervention to optimise bone and muscle health, and psychological assistance to address emotional and cognitive dimensions. The implementation of assistive technologies, such as walkers and wheelchairs, also plays a crucial role in improving patient autonomy. (G6mez Monedero, 2023).The approach and treatment of Immobility Syndrome in geriatric patients requires a multidisciplinary approach. Both pharmacological and non-pharmacological interventions must be implemented with the aim of improve mobility and prevent complications such as pressure ulcers, cognitive impairment and decreased cardiovascular and respiratory function. Non-pharmacological interventions include mobility exercises, physiotherapy, occupational therapy and adapted physical activity programmes. In terms of pharmacological interventions, medications can be used to relieve pain and inflammation, as well as nutritional supplements to improve overall health. It is essential to establish an individualised care plan that takes into account the needs and characteristics of each patient, promoting their autonomy and quality of life. In this sense, teamwork between doctors, nurses, physiotherapists, occupational therapists and other health professionals is essential. All of them must cooperate to provide comprehensive care to ensure the overall well-being of older patients.Patient and family education is also a crucial element in the management of Immobility Syndrome, as it allows them to understand the importance of following recommendations and actively participating in the patient's care. (Sanchez, 2023).

b. Fall Syndrome

Cafdas Syndrome is a common and serious condition in the geriatric population. It is defined as the occurrence of an unintentional caffeine attack resulting in physical, psychological or social injury.It is important to note that cauda equina can be considered as a symptom of an underlying medical problem or a consequence of the changes associated with ageing. The epidemiology of the cafdas syndrome shows a high prevalence in older adults and represents a significant cause of morbidity and mortality in this age group. Diagnosis of the caidas syndrome involves the assessment of risk factors and the identification of precipitating events. Assessment tools such as the Timed Up and Go (TUG) and Berg's Test are useful for assessing balance and gait, as well as other physical aspects related to cohabitation. The approach to and treatment of cauda equina syndrome include preventive and rehabilitative strategies, which are based on the identification and management of the specific risk factors present in each patient. Non-pharmacological interventions include physical exercise therapies,muscle strengthening and balance training programmes (Cedefio et al.2024) (Franco & Lisbeth, 2022) It is crucial for resident physicians to understand caffeine syndrome and to acquire the skills necessary for its diagnosis, management and prevention, as this will contribute to improving the quality of life and safety of older adults.

• Definition

Falls in the elderly population are defined as involuntary events that result in the person ending up on the floor or another lower level, without being the consequence of a major illness or a violent push. In geriatrics, falls are considered key indicators of frailty and increased risk of serious morbidities as well as decreased quality of life.

It is established by the presence of two or more unprovoked deaths in persons over 65 years of age in the last year.It is considered a very common condition in the geriatric population and represents a major public health problem due to the negative consequences it can have, such as fractures, functional disability and diminished quality of life.

Cafdas can be caused by multiple factors, including gait disturbances, muscle weakness, balance disorders and underlying medical conditions.

A comprehensive assessment is essential to identify the potential causes of the cystic fibrosis and to establish an individualised treatment plan that includes both pharmacological and non-pharmacological interventions to prevent recurrence of cystic fibrosis and improve patient safety and functionality (Cedefio et al.2024)(Tamayo Pérez, 2023).

• Epidemiology and Precipitating Factors

Cafdas Syndrome is a highly prevalent condition in older adults, being considered one of the main causes of disability and mortality in this population group. According to epidemiological studies, approximately 30% of adults over 65 years of age suffer at least one caffeine attack annually.

In addition, it is estimated that coffee is responsible for more than 50% of accidental injuries in people over 75 years of age. The consequences of the coffees can be severe, including hip fractures, head injuries and diminished quality of life. Importantly, this syndrome has a significant impact on health systems, generating high costs in terms of hospitalisations and medical care. Therefore, appropriate prevention and management strategies are essential to reduce the incidence of caffeine in this vulnerable population (Hart et al.2020)(Ganz & Latham, 2020).

Precipitating factors can be classified as intrinsic and extrinsic. Intrinsic factors include health problems such as muscle weakness, gait and balance disturbances, cognitive impairment and medication side effects. Extrinsic factors involve environmental conditions such as inadequate lighting, road obstacles and inappropriate footwear.

• Diagnosis and Assessment of the Elderly Patient at Risk of Cohabitation

The diagnosis of Fall Syndrome in older adults includes a thorough assessment to identify underlying causes and risk factors. This involves reviewing the patient's medical history, performing physical and functional tests, as well as examining the environmental conditions in which the individual is found. The assessment of an elderly patient at risk for cauda equina should be holistic and include a complete review of the medical history, physical examination and mobility testing. Tools such as the Berg Balance Scale and the Six Minute Gait Test are frequently used to assess cauda equina risk. These instruments can provide objective information about the risk of cauda equina and can detect deficits in balance and gait.

An accurate diagnosis will help to design a personalised treatment plan that includes interventions aimed at mitigating the identified risk factors and improving patient safety and mobility (Iglesias et al.2022). Particular attention should be paid to medication review and cognitive assessment, both of which can contribute significantly to the risk of coffees. (COLCHADO ROSALES, 2021).

• Preventive Interventions and Treatments

The approach and treatment of Cafdas Syndrome is based on several strategies. Initially, modifiable risk factors should be identified through a comprehensive assessment of the patient, including medical history, medications and other risk factors. The use of drugs, sensory and musculoskeletal disorders, among others, should be encouraged. Regular physical exercise should be encouraged, a balanced diet should be encouraged and muscles should be strengthened through specific training programmes.

In terms of techniques for preventing falls, measures such as removing obstacles in the environment, wearing appropriate footwear, using mobility aids and promoting safety in the home should be implemented.

Finally, it is essential to educate patients and their caregivers about strategies to prevent falls and how to act in case they occur. It is important to emphasise that the treatment of Cafdas Syndrome should be personalised, taking into account the needs and characteristics of each patient with the aim of reducing the risk of Cafdas and improving the quality of life.Interventions to prevent caffeine dependence in the elderly should be multifactorial and include adjustments to the home environment to eliminate risks, exercise programmes to improve strength and balance, and pharmacological screening to minimise side effects that may increase the risk of caffeine dependence. In addition, education on caffeine prevention is crucial for patients and caregivers. In some cases, assistive devices, such as canes or walkers, may be recommended to improve stability. (COLCHADO ROSALES, 2021).

c. Urinary Incontinence

Incontinence syndrome in the elderly is defined as the involuntary loss of urine that can affect the quality of life and autonomy of patients.

Epidemiology shows a high prevalence, especially in older women. Diagnosis involves assessment of medical history, physical examinations, laboratory tests and specific questionnaires to assess incontinence. Assessment tools include the pad test, the international incontinence severity scale, among others. The approach and treatment of incontinence in the older adult is multidisciplinary and includes lifestyle changes, pelvic floor exercises, containment devices, medications and in some cases, surgical procedures.

• Definition

Urinary incontinence is defined as the involuntary loss of urine, a common problem that significantly affects dignity and quality of life in the elderly population. This condition not only involves clinical, but also social and psychological distress, impacting on autonomy and participation in daily activities (Batmani et al., 2021) (Yagmur & Gül, 2021).

• Epidemiology of the incontinence syndrome in the elderly

Incontinence affects a large proportion of the geriatric population. According to studies, about 50% of people over 65 years of age have some degree of incontinence. Furthermore, it is estimated that 80% of cases of urinary incontinence occur in women. This information is crucial for the training of medical residents, as it enables them to understand the magnitude of the problem and the need to acquire skills for effective diagnosis and treatment in their clinical practice. (Gibson et al.2021).

• Types of Incontinence in the Elderly

In the elderly, urinary incontinence can be classified into several main types:

- Stress incontinence: urine leakage during coughing, sneezing or any activity that increases intra-abdominal pressure.
- Urge incontinence: urine leakage associated with a strong urge to urinate that is difficult to stop.
- Mixed incontinence: a combination of stress and urge incontinence.
- Overflow incontinence: occurs when the bladder does not empty completely, leading to frequent episodes of urination or continuous dribbling.

• Differential Diagnosis and Assessment

Diagnosis of Older Adult Incontinence Syndrome is crucial for proper treatment. It is necessary to use specific tools to assess urinary incontinence, such as symptom questionnaires, voiding diaries, pad tests, flowmetry, abdominal ultrasound, urodynamics, among others. It is also essential to take a detailed medical history, paying particular attention to medical and surgical history and current medication. The physical examination should include genital, urinary and neurological assessment. Additional tests such as urinalysis, microbiological culture, renal ultrasound, among others, should be considered to rule out other concurrent pathologies. Urodynamic evaluations may be necessary to differentiate between types of incontinence and to rule out other underlying medical conditions. It is essential to consider factors such as medications, comorbidities and cognitive impairment, which may influence the presentation and management of incontinence (Shaw & Wagg, 2021). Timely diagnosis will allow a comprehensive and personalised management plan to be established for each patient, taking into account factors such as the underlying cause, severity, impact on quality of life and therapeutic goals". (Radoja and Degmecié2020) (Nambiar et al.2022)

• Valuation Instruments

In the context of older adult incontinence, assessment instruments are a crucial part of the diagnostic process. Some of the most commonly used instruments include the Urinary Incontinence Questionnaire (ICIQ), the Incontinence Assessment Questionnaire (IAQ) and the Incontinence Severity Scale (IS). (Radoja and Degmecié.2020). These instruments allow resident physicians to collect detailed information on the frequency, severity and impact of incontinence on patients' daily lives. In addition, they facilitate the identification of possible underlying causes and contribute to the formulation of an appropriate and personalised treatment plan for each patient, which is essential in the comprehensive management of this geriatric syndrome" (O'Connor et al.2021). (O'Connor et al.2021)

• Treatment Options and Multidisciplinary Management

Treatment of urinary incontinence in the elderly should be individualised and may include:

- Behavioural modifications: such as bladder training and pelvic floor strengthening exercises.
- Pharmacotherapy: medicines specific according to on type of incontinence.
- Minimally invasive interventions: such as botulinum toxin injections or intravaginal devices.
- Surgery: in selected cases where other therapies have not been effective.

This management requires the collaboration of a multidisciplinary team including urologists, geriatricians, specialist nurses, physiotherapists, and psychologists, ensuring comprehensive and patient-centred care.

d. Cognitive Impairment

Cognitive Impairment Syndrome is characterised by a decline in cognitive skills, such as memory, language, attention and reasoning, which affects a person's ability to carry out daily activities.This syndrome is more common in older people and can be caused by different conditions, such as Alzheimer's disease or vascular dementia. The prevalence of cognitive impairment syndrome increases with age and is estimated to affect about 20% of adults over 65 years of age. Diagnosis of the syndrome is based on clinical assessment, patient history and neuropsychological testing. Some of the assessment instruments used include the Mini-Mental State Examination (MMSE) and the Montreal Cognitive Assessment (MoCA). Management and treatment of this syndrome include pharmacological and non-pharmacological interventions, such as medications to improve cognitive function, occupational therapy and cognitive stimulation programmes.

It is essential for resident physicians to acquire the necessary knowledge about this syndrome in order to make an accurate diagnosis and provide appropriate treatment to their patients.

• Definition and Epidemiology

Cognitive Impairment Syndrome is defined as a set of cognitive and functional symptoms affecting memory, language, attention, reasoning and the ability to perform activities of daily living.

These symptoms have a gradual and progressive onset and often interfere significantly with the independence and quality of life of older people. This syndrome is not a disease in itself, but can be caused by a variety of conditions such as Alzheimer's disease, vascular dementia and other neurodegenerative diseases. A comprehensive assessment including neuropsychological tests and rating scales is essential to establish an accurate diagnosis... (Chorefio-Parra et al.2020)(Parada et al.2022). The epidemiology of Cognitive Impairment Syndrome is of great relevance to understand the prevalence and impact of this condition in the geriatric population. According to epidemiological studies, it is estimated that about 10-20% of older adults suffer from some degree of cognitive impairment, which is a risk factor for dementia. In addition, older age and the presence of certain chronic diseases, such as hypertension and diabetes, have been found to increase the likelihood of developing dementia. These data highlight the importance of adequately addressing the diagnosis and treatment of Cognitive Impairment Syndrome in resident physicians, in order to improve the quality of life of geriatric patients and reduce the burden that this condition imposes on health systems. (Fonte Sevillano & Santos Hedman, 2020) (Parada et al., 2022).

As the world's population ages, the impact of cognitive impairment continues to grow, representing a significant challenge for both health systems and the families of those affected.

• Classification and Aetiology of Cognitive Impairment

Cognitive impairment can be classified into two main categories: mild cognitive impairment (MCI) and dementia. MCI is characterised by cognitive decline that does not significantly interfere with daily activities, while dementia involves a loss of cognitive function sufficient to interfere with the individual's independence. The causes of cognitive decline are varied, including genetic factors, neurological diseases such as Alzheimer's disease and vascular dementia, and modifiable risk factors such as hypertension, diabetes, high cholesterol, lack of exercise and poor diet. In addition, psychosocial factors such as social isolation and depression may also contribute to the development of cognitive decline.

• Cognitive Assessment Tools

The diagnosis of Cognitive Impairment Syndrome is made by a comprehensive assessment including neuropsychological testing, clinical assessment and interviews with the patient and caregivers. Specific assessment instruments such as the Mini-Mental State Examination (MMSE) and the Clinical Dementia Rating (CDR) are used to measure the degree of cognitive impairment. In addition, neuroimaging tests, such as brain MRI, may be performed to rule out other causes of cognitive impairment. It is important to bear in mind that the diagnosis should be made by a trained physician, based on a structured assessment, as Cognitive Impairment Syndrome can be associated with different types of dementia, such as Alzheimer's disease. (Cancino et al.2020).

An early and accurate diagnosis will allow the establishment of appropriate management and treatment strategies to improve the quality of life of patients and their caregivers (Galvez, 2024)(Parada et al.2022).

Several neuropsychological tools and tests are used to diagnose and assess cognitive impairment. These include:

- Mini-Mental State Examination (MMSE)**: a brief test used to assess cognitive function.
- Montreal Cognitive Assessment (MoCA)**: designed to identify MCI and mild dementia.
- Clock Test: a simple and effective test for assessing executive and visuospatial function.
- In addition, questionnaires such as the Informant Questionnaire on Cognitive Decline in the Elderly (IQCODE) can be used to obtain additional information from patients' informants.

These instruments allow for an objective and quantitative assessment of cognitive impairment, which facilitates accurate diagnosis and treatment monitoring. It is important that resident physicians become familiar with these instruments and learn to use them correctly in order to perform a complete and accurate assessment of patients with Cognitive Impairment Syndrome (Valenzuela Sanchez & Marcelino Arias, 2023) (Quinaloa et al.2020).The choice of the appropriate tool depends on the clinical situation and the degree of impairment suspected. These assessments should be complemented by clinical analyses and, in some cases, brain imaging tests to rule out other causes of the symptoms.

• Patient Care and Management Strategies

The approach and treatment of Cognitive Impairment Syndrome is based on a comprehensive assessment of the cognitive functions and general health status of the geriatric patient. (Garcfa-Ribas et al.2023). The main objective is to slow cognitive decline and improve the patient's quality of life. The approach and treatment of Cognitive Impairment Syndrome involves pharmacological and non-pharmacological strategies, such as cognitive stimulation, occupational therapy and emotional support, with the aim of improving patients' quality of life and delaying the progression of symptoms. The use of anticholinesterase drugs to improve cognitive symptoms should be considered.

The management of cognitive impairment involves a multidisciplinary approach that includes doctors, nurses, therapists and social workers. Interventions may include:

- Medical management: adjustment of medications that may exacerbate cognitive impairment and use of drugs to treat specific symptoms or to slow the progression of dementia.
- Psychosocial interventions: such as cognitive stimulation therapies, group activities, and emotional support for both patient and caregivers.
- Environmental modifications: ensuring that the patient's living environment is safe and stimulating.

Teamwork with other health professionals, such as psychologists and therapists, is essential to provide comprehensive care tailored to the needs of each patient. It is also necessary to provide information and support to caregivers and family members, as they play a crucial role in the daily management and care of the patient with Cognitive Impairment Syndrome (Sailema Lalaleo, 2023) (Mazo Bafiol & Moncada Botero, 2023).

e. Sarcopenia

Sarcopenia is a geriatric syndrome characterised by progressive and generalised loss of muscle mass, strength and function, and is associated with an increased risk of disability, disability and impaired quality of life in the older population.

It is estimated to affect approximately 10% of adults over 60 years of age and its prevalence increases with age. Diagnosis is based on clinical assessment of muscle strength and function, as well as laboratory tests to rule out other causes of weakness. The approach and treatment of sarcopenia focuses on multidisciplinary interventions including physical exercise, nutritional therapy and risk factor management. It is essential that resident physicians acquire knowledge of sarcopenia and its management in order to identify and appropriately manage this condition in the geriatric population. (Pérez Carvajal, 2023)(Sandoval Animas).

• Definition and Pathophysiological Mechanisms

Sarcopenia is characterised as a progressive and generalised decline in skeletal muscle mass and muscle function, which is associated with an increased risk of adverse outcomes such as disability, fractures, physical dependence and mortality. From a pathophysiological point of view, sarcopenia is the result of an imbalance between muscle protein synthesis and muscle protein degradation, a process influenced by factors such as ageing, physical inactivity, systemic inflammation, malnutrition, and endocrine disruption.

• Epidemiology

It is one of the most important areas of study in relation to geriatric syndromes. It is estimated that the prevalence of sarcopenia in adults over 60 years of age varies between 5% and 25%, depending on the diagnostic criteria used. Furthermore, it has been observed that sarcopenia tends to increase with age, being more common in people over 80 years of age. This condition is associated with a number of risk factors, such as lack of physical activity, malnutrition, inflammation and chronic diseases such as diabetes and chronic obstructive pulmonary disease (Petermann-Rocha et al.2022)(Gao et al., 2021)(Almohaisen et al.2022).

• Diagnosis according to EWGSOP2

The most recent update of the European Working Group on Sarcopenia in Older People (EWGSOP2) proposes a practical and sequential approach to the diagnosis of sarcopenia, focusing initially on risk detection by gait speed. A gait pace of less than 0.8 m/s suggests sarcopenia, which should be followed by measurement of grip strength and assessment of muscle mass to confirm the diagnosis. Grip strength is considered low when it is less than 27 kg for men and 16 kg for women. Muscle mass, assessed by methods such as dual energy X-ray absorptiometry (DEXA) or electrical bioimpedance, also provides quantitative criteria for diagnostic confirmation (Moretti et al.2024).

• Current Diagnostic Methods and Criteria

In addition to DEXA and bioimpedance, other imaging techniques such as computed tomography (CT) and magnetic resonance imaging (MRI) can be used for a detailed assessment of body composition. These methods allow not only to identify the reduction of muscle mass, but also to analyse the quality of muscle tissue, including fat infiltration and fibrosis. The implementation of of these criteria and methods allows for an accurate and differentiated diagnosis of the sarcopenia, facilitating more effective interventions (Loyola et al.2020) (Criollo Sanchez, 2024).

• Therapeutic Approaches and Prevention

The approach and treatment of sarcopenia is based on a combination of pharmacological and non-pharmacological interventions. Treatment is based on 2 main pillars: protein-rich diets (mainly leucine and HMB), and resistance-power training with the aim of promoting an increase in muscle mass and strength.Nutritional supplements should also be provided in case of protein and vitamin D deficiencies.It is important to encourage regular physical activity, such as walking or balance exercises, to improve muscle function. Other non-pharmacological approaches include occupational therapy to facilitate independence in daily activities and physiotherapy to improve mobility. As for pharmacological interventions, there is currently no effective strategy to improve muscle mass or quality, it is important to evaluate the potential risks and benefits before initiating any pharmacological treatment in geriatric patients (Barajas-Galindo et al.2021)(Murri, 2021).

**f.**Fragility

Frailty syndrome is a common condition in older adults and is characterised by decreased physiological reserve and increased vulnerability to stress. It is defined as a medical condition characterised by the presence of weakness, reduced walking speed, decreased physical activity, unintentional weight loss and decreased cognitive function. Frailty affects approximately 10-25% of people over 65 years of age and the prevalence increases with age. The diagnosis of frailty is based on clinical criteria, which may include the Fried frailty scale and the Rockwood frailty index. The approach and treatment of frailty involves multidisciplinary interventions including physical exercise, optimisation of physical activity and exercise therapy. nutrition, medication management, cognitive therapy and risk factor reduction (Kaçmaz et al., 2023)(Montesino et al.2022). It is essential that resident physicians are trained in the recognition and management of this syndrome in order to provide quality care to geriatric patients.

• Definition

Frailty is defined as a state of increased vulnerability to external stressors, due to a decrease in physiological reserves in the body.
multiple body systems. This syndrome is characteristic of the elderly population and is associated with an elevated risk of adverse events such as disability, hospitalisation and mortality. (Barillas Escobar & Henrfquez Mezquita, 2021).

• Epidemiology

Frailty Syndrome is a common geriatric problem worldwide, especially affecting people over 65 years of age. It is estimated that between 4% and 27% of community-dwelling older adults and up to 50% of residents in geriatric institutions have frailty. Moreover, the prevalence of frailty increases with age, being higher in women (Martfnez et al., 2024).

Frailty is also associated with increased morbidity and mortality, as well as increased health care utilisation. These data demonstrate the importance of adequately addressing and treating this syndrome in resident physicians in order to provide comprehensive care and improve the quality of life of geriatric patients (Martfnez et al., 2024).

• Conceptualisation and Relevance in Geriatrics

In geriatrics, frailty is recognised as a key predictor of health outcomes in older adults and a critical factor in planning their care. Its relevance lies in its ability to identify individuals at high risk of rapid deterioration, allowing the implementation of specific preventive and therapeutic strategies that can significantly improve their prognosis and quality of life.

• Fragility Assessment Models (G6mez Monedero, 2023)(L6pez, 2023)

There are several models for assessing frailty, two of which stand out:

- Fried's Phenotypic Model: This model identifies frailty by the presence of five criteria: unintentional weight loss, weakness (as measured by grip strength), exhaustion, slowness and low level of physical activity. The presence of three or more of these criteria classifies an individual as frail.
- Cumulative Frailty Index: This approach views frailty as an accumulation of deficits over time, assessing a wide range of variables including symptoms, signs, diseases, disabilities and laboratory findings. A greater number of deficits is associated with more severe frailty.

• Impact of Fragility

The impact of frailty in the elderly population is profound, affecting not only physical health but also autonomy and social interaction. Frail individuals are more likely to suffer from impaired quality of life, increased use of health services, and increased dependence on long-term care. In addition, frailty may exacerbate the course of other chronic diseases, complicating their management and treatment.

• Interventions to Enhance Resilience and Quality of Life

The approach and treatment of Frailty Syndrome in geriatric patients focuses on comprehensive and multidimensional care.

It is essential to design a care plan that addresses the risk factors and underlying causes of frailty. This implies an interdisciplinary approach that includes specific actions to improve patients' physical, nutritional and cognitive functioning.

Non-pharmacological interventions include personalised physical exercise, occupational therapy, cognitive stimulation and adequate nutrition. In terms of pharmacological treatment, different medications can be used to manage comorbidities and symptoms associated with frailty. In addition, it is essential to provide a safe environment adapted to the patient's needs, as well as social and emotional support to improve quality of life. Interventions to manage frailty focus on improving the individual's resilience and functional capacity. These include:

- Physical exercise programmes: Designed to improve strength, balance and general endurance.
- Nutritional optimisation: Ensuring a diet rich in protein, vitamins and minerals essential for maintaining muscle mass and immune function.
- Integrated chronic disease management: Coordinating care between different specialists to optimise the treatment of co-morbidities.
- Psychosocial support: Providing social and psychological assistance to promote social inclusion and combat depression and loneliness.

3. Multidisciplinary Approach to Geriatric Syndromes

The multidisciplinary approach to geriatric syndromes is essential to provide comprehensive care to patients. This approach involves a variety of health professionals, such as geriatric physicians, nurses, physiotherapists, occupational therapists and social workers, among others. Each professional brings specific expertise and knowledge to assess and treat geriatric syndromes from different perspectives. Teamwork allows for a comprehensive assessment of patients, considering medical as well as social, psychological and functional dimensions. Effective communication is established between the different specialists involved, which facilitates shared decision-making and treatment coordination. This improves the quality of life of geriatric patients and reduces complications and hospitalisations. This multidisciplinary approach is especially relevant in geriatric syndromes, as these are often multifactorial and require a holistic approach that considers all dimensions of the older person. Teamwork also allows for a more comprehensive view of the patient's health, as each professional can detect aspects that others may miss, resulting in a more effective and personalised treatment for each individual. Multidisciplinary collaboration provides comprehensive support to patients and their families, addressing not only medical, but also emotional, social and lifestyle needs. In short, the multidisciplinary approach in the treatment of geriatric syndromes represents a holistic and effective way to improve the quality of life and well-being of older people.

4. Pharmacological and Non-pharmacological Treatment Pharmacological Treatment

The treatment of geriatric syndromes is approached both pharmacological and non-pharmacological. In the case of pharmacological treatment, medications are used to address the symptoms and underlying causes of geriatric syndromes. For example, in immobility syndrome, medications may be prescribed for pain and inflammation, as well as to improve mobility. In the case of non-pharmacological treatment, non-drug interventions and therapies are used. These may include physical and occupational therapy, exercise programmes, dietary changes and adaptation of the physical environment. Cognitive and emotional therapy techniques may also be used to address geriatric syndromes such as cognitive impairment and frailty. In general, pharmacological and non-pharmacological treatment are used in a complementary manner to optimise the management of geriatric syndromes and improve the quality of life of older patients.

5. Importance of Training in Geriatric Syndromes for Physicians Residents

Training in geriatric syndromes is of utmost importance for resident physicians due to the increasing ageing of the population and the growing demand for medical care in this patient group.

Geriatric syndromes are common clinical conditions in older adults and their proper management requires specific knowledge and clinical skills. These syndromes, such as immobility, coffee, cognitive impairment, sarcopenia and frailty, are associated with an increased risk of disability, hospitalisation, institutionalisation and mortality.

Lack of adequate training in geriatric syndromes can lead to inadequate diagnosis and treatment, as well as increased complications. and negative patient outcomes. It is therefore essential that resident physicians acquire the knowledge and skills necessary to identify and manage these syndromes in a comprehensive manner, providing optimal and quality care for older adults.

Particular attention should be paid to the importance of appropriate drug management in older patients, as inappropriate pharmacotherapy may increase the risk of drug-drug interactions and adverse effects. It is essential to promote continuing education in geriatric syndromes to ensure that resident physicians are trained to provide quality, comprehensive care to the growing population of older adults.

6. B-learning in the Teaching of Geriatric Syndromes

B-learning is an innovative methodology that effectively combines face-to-face and online learning to facilitate the teaching of Geriatric Symptoms to resident doctors. This educational strategy is based on the use of digital and technological resources to allow students to access theoretical content, case studies, videos and other educational resources from any location and at any time. It encourages active participation through discussion forums, collaborative activities and online assessments, promoting the acquisition of theoretical and practical knowledge, as well as the development of clinical skills and informed decision making in the approach and treatment of Geriatric Symptoms.By combining face-to-face and online teaching, B-Learning offers flexibility and adaptability to the individual needs of resident doctors, allowing them to access content autonomously and develop their learning at their own pace. This methodology provides a more enriching and effective learning experience, improving knowledge retention and skills transfer to clinical practice. In summary, B-learning is an innovative educational strategy that optimises the teaching of Geriatric Symptoms to resident physicians, providing them with state-of-the-art learning tools and resources to enhance their training and professional performance. The B-learning method helps doctorsThe programme is designed to enable residents to acquire technical skills and theoretical knowledge in a flexible and adaptable way to meet their individual needs.This innovative methodology is highly effective and enriching, allowing resident doctors to develop their skills at their own pace and in any location. The B-learning approach encourages active participation through discussion forums and collaborative activities, allowing students to learn in a more holistic manner. Thanks to the combination of face-to-face and online learning, resident doctors can significantly improve their training and professional performance.

a. Methodologies and Tools of B-learning

In the teaching of Geriatric Symptoms to medical residents through B-learning, various methodologies and tools can be used to support the teaching-learning process. The methodologies include a combination of face-to-face and virtual classes, allowing flexibility in time and space for learning. In addition, techniques such as clinical case studies, virtual simulations and debates are used, encouraging the active participation of students and the application of theoretical knowledge in real situations. This is done through the use of technological tools such as educational platforms and interactive multimedia resources, which facilitate access to study material, feedback and assessment of learning.These B-learning methodologies and tools contribute to improve the training of resident doctors in geriatric disorders, promoting a more dynamic, participative and student-centred learning.

b. Content Design for Teaching Geriatric Syndromes in B-learning

The design of content for teaching geriatric syndromes in b-learning is essential to ensure effective learning. It is important to define The objectives of each module, as well as the contents to be covered, must be clearly and concisely stated. It should be taken into account that B-learning combines face-to-face teaching with online learning, so it is necessary to adapt the materials and teaching strategies to this modality. For this purpose, various resources such as interactive presentations, educational videos, case studies and discussion forums can be used. It is essential to establish a logical and coherent sequence in the presentation of content so that Resident doctors can acquire knowledge in a progressive manner. Assessment activities should be included to measure the level of understanding and retention of information. In summary, the design of content for teaching geriatric syndromes in B-learning should be didactic, interactive and adapted to the needs of the resident physicians.

i. Design Methodologies

In the teaching of geriatric symptoms to medical residents through B-learning, design methodologies play a key role.

1. Virtual Forums

Virtual forums are a form of online interaction that allows resident physicians to discuss and share ideas about geriatric syndromes. These forums provide a virtual space where participants can ask questions, raise and respond to comments, and share relevant resources (Fernandez et al.2022).Virtual forums encourage active participation and knowledge sharing among resident physicians, which facilitates collaborative learning and the development of skills in the management and treatment of geriatric syndromes.

They allow interaction with experts in the field, who can provide guidance and advice (Sanchez et al.2023).In this sense, virtual forums are an effective tool to promote discussion and learning among resident physicians in the context of B-learning; they are an essential tool for information exchange and collaboration among physicians from different specialties, which contributes significantly to the advancement of geriatric medicine. The possibility of fluid conversations through virtual platforms allows health professionals to access different perspectives, discover new practices and improve their clinical skills in order to provide optimal care to patients.geriatric patients. The flexibility and ease of access to virtual forums allows physicians to keep up to date on relevant topics and to participate in the development of new research and the implementation of best practices in the care of elderly patients. (Céspedes-Tamayo et al.2020).

In summary, virtual forums represent a valuable tool for the strengthening of the medical community and the continuous improvement of geriatric care.

2. Virtual Simulation

Virtual simulation is a methodology used in the teaching of geriatric disorders to medical residents. It involves the use of virtual reality software and technology to recreate realistic clinical situations and allow students to practice and acquire skills in a safe and controlled environment.Through virtual simulation, resident doctors can be confronted with complex clinical cases and apply their theoretical knowledge in medical decision-making. This methodology also allows them to receive immediate feedback, which encourages active learning and continuous improvement.Virtual simulation offers the advantage of being flexible in terms of time and place of study, as it can be done individually and at different times.

This teaching methodology is particularly useful for the acquisition of practical clinical skills and the development of competencies necessary in the management and treatment of geriatric syndromes. The use of virtual simulation enables resident physicians to improve their ability to effectively diagnose and treat geriatric patients. By providing a realistic and safe environment, residents can practice in scenarios that mimic the complexity and challenges of medical care for the elderly. This gives them the opportunity to apply their knowledge in a controlled environment and receive immediate feedback on their decisions. (Siew et al., 2021).

Virtual simulation also allows them to learn how to manage highly complex clinical situations, which is crucial for their training as physicians. Moreover, by being able to perform simulation at flexible times and locations, resident physicians can tailor their education to their own needs and responsibilities (Chaby et al.2022). In summary, virtual simulation is a valuable tool for the training of medical residents in the management of geriatric syndromes, providing a safe, effective and flexible way to acquire and improve clinical skills.

3. Inverted classroom

The inverted classroom is a teaching methodology that promotes active learning and the participation of resident doctors. In this modality, students study the theoretical contents of geriatric syndromes autonomously before class, using didactic materials such as videos, readings or online tutorials. Subsequently, in the classroom, discussion, case analysis and practical problem solving are encouraged, which facilitates the application of the knowledge acquired. This strategy makes better use of class time and promotes deeper learning, as the resident doctors can resolve doubts and receive direct feedback from the teacher.By carrying out practical activities in groups, teamwork and collaboration among participants are encouraged, which are essential skills in the management of geriatric syndromes. The flipped classroom creates a collaborative learning environment that empowers residents to develop complex and critical cognitive skills. Knowledge construction is encouraged through debate and discussion, allowing residents to analyse and reflect on learning material from different perspectives. The model also encourages individual resident responsibility in the learning process by promoting prior preparation and active participation in classroom activities. This methodology also fosters the development of effective communication skills, teaching residents to express their ideas clearly and coherently. (Masud et al.2022)(Ong et al.2021)(Wu et al., 2020)

In summary, the flipped classroom is an effective technique for teaching about these syndromes, as it encourages active learning, participation and teamwork of the medical residents. In short, the flipped classroom is a powerful tool for improving the quality of medical education through the active participation of residents and the promotion of meaningful and collaborative learning. The flipped classroom enriches the educational experience by promoting constructive discussion that empowers residents to analyse and reflect on geriatric syndromes from a variety of perspectives. Also, the model fosters critical and autonomous inquiry, encouraging residents to engage actively with their learning process and to actively seek understanding and mastery of the content.

4. Asynchronous Class

The asynchronous classroom is a teaching methodology used in B-learning that allows resident doctors to access materials and content in a flexible and autonomous manner. In this modality, participants can access videos, readings, and other online resources at their own pace, giving them the opportunity to review content and delve deeper into topics of interest. (Wu et al., 2020).It encourages interaction between resident physicians through virtual forums and other online communication tools, where they can discuss and resolve questions. This approach allows residents to tailor their learning to their own needs and schedules, which promotes greater participation and understanding in the study of geriatric syndromes. The flexibility of the asynchronous classroom also facilitates access to continuing medical education, as it allows residents to continue learning despite work and personal obligations. (Ong et al.2021)In summary, this methodology encourages autonomy and responsibility in the learning process, preparing resident doctors for a more reflective professional practice committed to constant updating of medical knowledge.

5. Virtual Tutoring

Virtual tutoring is a fundamental tool in the B-learning of geriatric syndromes. Through this modality, resident doctors can receive guidance, support and follow-up from tutors who are experts in the field.During the virtual tutorials, residents can ask questions, receive feedback on their clinical cases and discuss approach and treatment strategies. These sessions allow for the joint review of assessment tools used in the diagnosis of geriatric syndromes.Virtual tutoring encourages autonomous learning and interaction between tutors and residents, promoting a space for reflection and analysis of real cases. Likewise, This type of tutoring facilitates access to up-to-date information and relevant bibliographic resources (Masud et al.2022).

Virtual mentoring also allows them to develop communication and collaboration skills through virtual platforms, which is essential in today's healthcare environment. In addition, by fostering resident autonomy, virtual mentoring gives residents a greater sense of responsibility and control over their learning. Expert tutors can share relevant clinical experiences and case studies, which enriches residents' training and provides them with a practical perspective that complements their clinical training (Ong et al.2021)(Pan et al., 2024). Through virtual tutoring, specialised training sessions and keynote lectures by opinion leaders in the field of geriatrics can be accessed. In summary, virtual tutoring is an effective pedagogical strategy to strengthen the knowledge and skills of resident physicians in the management of geriatric syndromes through direct interaction with experts in the field that promotes the professional development of residents and helps them to keep up to date with the latest trends and advances in the treatment of geriatric syndromes.

c. Experiences in Medical Education

In the field of medical education, various experiences have been developed in the teaching of geriatric syndromes through the use of the B-learning modality. These experiences have focused on providing resident doctors with the opportunity to broaden their knowledge of the different geriatric syndromes, as well as providing them with practical tools for their approach and treatment, enabling them to acquire the skills and competencies necessary to provide comprehensive and quality care to geriatric patients. (Stefanowicz-Kocol et al., 2023).However, limitations have also been identified in the implementation of B-learning in medical education, such as lack of access to technological resources, resistance to change or difficulty in assessing learning in virtual environments. (Piot et al.2020).Despite these challenges, successful experiences in the teaching of geriatric disorders with a B-learning approach represent an opportunity to improve the training of resident doctors and to guarantee adequate care for the geriatric population.

i. Expectations and Limitations

Regarding the expectations of B-learning in the teaching of geriatric syndromes to medical residents, it is expected that this methodology will provide a flexible and accessible environment for learning, allowing students to access the content at any time and place.

The use of virtual tools and interaction with other students and tutors in virtual forums is expected to promote greater engagement and active participation in the learning process. However, it is important to consider the limitations of this methodology, such as the need for access to the internet and technological devices, as well as the possibility that some students may have difficulties adapting to this form of learning. It should also be borne in mind that B-learning requires careful planning to ensure the effective integration of the different learning components and activities.

d. Learning Assessment in Geriatric Syndromes with a B-learning Approach

The assessment of learning in geriatric disorders with a B-learning approach is essential to measure the knowledge acquired by resident doctors.Different assessment strategies should be used, such as written tests, case studies, practical activities and continuous assessment.The B-learning approach provides the opportunity to assess both the theoretical knowledge and practical skills of the residents. In addition, it is important to evaluate the learning process in geriatric syndromes, identifying the strengths and weaknesses of the residents, in order to provide adequate feedback and to continuously improve the teaching.

Assessment must be objective, fair and based on established criteria in order to ensure quality and academic rigour in the training of medical residents.

e. Successful and Good Experiences

Practice in the Teaching of Geriatric Syndromes with B-learning In the teaching of Geriatric Symptoms with B-learning, several successful experiences and good practices have been identified. Some of them include the integration of real and relevant clinical cases so that resident doctors can apply their theoretical knowledge in practical situations.

The use of interactive virtual platforms, where residents can access study materials, carry out activities and participate in discussion forums with other professionals, has also been found to be beneficial (Siew et al., 2021).

It is important to have a multidisciplinary teaching team that provides personalised support and feedback to residents (Masud et al.2022). These successful experiences and good practices have allowed to improve the learning and training of resident doctors in the approach and treatment of Geriatric Syndromes from the B-learning approach.

## f.Challenges and Opportunities in the Implementation of B-Learning in the Teaching of Geriatric Syndromes

The implementation of B-learning in the teaching of geriatric disorders presents a number of challenges and opportunities.

One of the challenges is the adaptation of traditional content and methodologies to a B-learning format, which combines face-to-face and online learning. This requires reviewing and adjusting teaching materials to ensure that they are accessible and effective in both physical and virtual environments.

Educators need to be trained in the use of the technological tools and resources necessary to implement B-learning successfully. The implementation of B-learning also offers significant opportunities. Through B-learning, resident physicians can access a variety of online resources, such as videos, case studies and simulations, that enrich their learning process. Online learning allows for the adaptation of the time and pace of study of each resident, enhancing their autonomy and self-discipline.

In summary, the implementation of B-learning in the teaching of geriatric disorders poses challenges in terms of adaptation and training, but also offers opportunities to improve the accessibility and quality of learning for resident doctors.

## 7. Conclusions and Recommendations for Teaching Geriatric Syndromes to Resident Physicians

In conclusion, the teaching of geriatric syndromes to medical residents is of vital importance to prepare health professionals in the comprehensive management of the elderly population.

It is essential that resident physicians acquire a sound knowledge of the definition, concepts, epidemiology, characteristics, approach and treatment of the different geriatric syndromes, such as immobility, cohabitation, cognitive impairment, sarcopenia and frailty. This will enable them to offer quality care, based on scientific evidence and adapted to the particular needs of geriatric patients. Therefore, it is recommended to include specific content on geriatric syndromes in the training programmes of resident doctors, as well as to use B-learning methodologies and tools to optimise the teaching-learning process.

It is essential to encourage a multidisciplinary approach and the use of both pharmacological and non-pharmacological approaches in the treatment of these syndromes. I consider it important to share successful experiences and best practices among health professionals in order to generate knowledge and improve the quality of teaching in this field. Despite the challenges and opportunities presented by the implementation of B-learning in the teaching of geriatric disorders, further progress in this direction is essential to train competent resident physicians committed to the care of the geriatric population.

## REFERENCES


• Pefia, K. P., Morera, M. R., Chaves, F. O., Quir6s, K. V. L., & Quir6s, S. L. (2020). Geriatric syndromes: coffee, incontinence and cognitive impairment. Revista Hispanoamericana de Ciencias de la Salud (RHCS), 6(4), 201-210. unirioja.es

• Corzo Camacho, M. A. (). Construcci6n de un m6dulo educativo para la ensefianza de los grandes sfndromes geriatricos por medio del uso de aprendizaje basado en problemas y tecnologfas .. repositorio.unal.edu.co. unal.edu.co.

• Tamayo Pérez, L. (2023). Fragility and geriatric syndromes in a group of institutionalised elderly people. uva.es

• Suarez Tomala, G. A. (2022). Deterioration of physical mobility and its influence on the psychological well-being of older adults. Basti6n Popular type C health centre. Guayaquil, 2022. upse.edu.ec

• Cuasapaz-Bermeo, A. E., Davas-Torres, C. C., Granda-Carbo, M. V., Zambrano-Santana, J. P., & Ponce-Alencastro, J. A. (2023). Clinical assessment and follow-up of pressure ulcers in geriatric patients: An integrated review of the literature. Multidisciplinary & Health Education Journal, 5(2), 279-285. journalmhe.org.

• MUNOZ, D. Y. S. (). . OF SOCIODEMOGRAPHIC, CLINICAL AND FUNCTIONAL CAPACITY VARIABLES WITH THE RISK OF FALLS IN ADULTS. MAYORS OF THE MUNICIPALITY OF ... core.ac.uk. core.ac.uk

• Sanchez, A. (2023). Abordaje kinésico domiciliario en patologfas del adulto mayor. ufasta.edu.ar

• G6mez Monedero, A. (2023). Aproximaci6n a los instrumentos de evaluación del sfundrome de fragilidad: scoping review. universidadeuropea.com.

• Cedefio, K. O. C., Narvaez, E. R. C., Contreras, J. N. I., & Ortiz, B. D. G. (2024). Polyneuropsychopharmacy: Updated Review of its Complications in the Geriatric Population. Ciencia Latina Revista Cientffica Multidisciplinar, 8(1), 1759-1775. ciencialatina.org.

• Franco, F. & Lisbeth, G. (2022). Factores de riesgo de cafda en los adultos mayores del barrio Parafso, parroquia Anconcito 2022... upse.edu.ec

• Hart, L. A., Phelan, E. A., Yi, J. Y., Marcum, Z. A., & Gray, S. L. (2020). Use of fall risk-increasing drugs around a fall-related injury in older adults: A systematic review. Journal of the American Geriatrics Society, 68(6), 1334- 1343. nih.gov.

• Ganz, D. A. & Latham, N. K. (2020). Prevention of falls in community-dwelling older adults. New England journal of medicine. escholarship.org

• Iglesias, A. L., Sanchez, L. H., Mateos-Nozal, J., & Nebreda, M. Â. (2022). Cafdas and hip fracture. Medicine-Programa de Formaci6n Médica Continuada Acreditado, 13(62), 3659-3670.

• COLCHADO ROSALES, B. (2021). Efectividad de ejercicios de coordinaci6n y equilibrio en la marcha del adulto mayor en un Hospital Publico, Chimbote 2019. usanpedro.edu.pe

• Chorefio-Parra, J. A., De la Rosa-Arredondo, T., & Guadarrama-Ortfz, P. (2020).

Abordaje diagn6stico del paciente con deterioro cognitivo en el primer nivel de atenci6n. Med Int Méx, 36(6). utel.edu.mx
• Parada Mufioz, K. R., Guapizaca Juca, J. F., & Bueno Pacheco, G. A. (2022). Cognitive impairment and depression in older adults: a systematic review of the last 5 years. Revista Cientffica UISRAEL, 9(2), 77-93. senescyt.gob.ec
• Fonte Sevillano, T. & Santos Hedman, D. J. (2020). Mild cognitive impairment in people over 85 years old. Cuban journal of medicine. sld.cu.
• Galvez, C. M. G. (2024). Usefulness of the STROOP test in the evaluation of cognitive functions in people with dementia. CIENCIAMATRIA. unirioja.es
• Valenzuela Sanchez, E. J. & Marcelino Arias, N. K. (2023). . Correlation between the cognitive impairment identified in the mini-mental state examination test and the diagnostic criteria for Alzheimer's disease in the hospital.unphu.edu.do
• Quinaloa, J. G. L., Guamangate, Y. K. M., Caisaluisa, J. L. M., & Cerda, V. D. C. T. (2020). Minimental test for early diagnosis of cognitive impairment. INNOVA Research Journal, 5(3), 13. unirioja.es
• Cancino, M., Rehbein, L., G6mez-Pérez, D., & Ortiz, M. S. (2020). Assessment of cognitive functioning in adults: Analysis and contrast of three of the most widely used instruments in Chile. Revista médica de Chile, 148(4), 452-458. scielo.cl
• Sailema Lalaleo, A. J. (2023). Gufa de estimulaci6n cognitiva y su efecto en adultos mayores con deterioro cognitivo. uta.edu.ec
• Mazo Bafiol, Y. & Moncada Botero, M. (2023). Protocolo de estimulaci6n cognitiva de las funciones ejecutivas en adultos mayores con demencia por cuerpos de Lewy. ces.edu.co
• Garcfa-Ribas, G., Marfn, A. S., & Barreto, P. L. (2023). Treatment of cognitive impairment. Medicine-Programa de Formaci6n Médica Continuada Acreditado, 13(74), 4382-4394.
• Radoja, I., & Degmecié, D. (2020). Urinary incontinence: diagnostic evaluation and first-line treatment. Southeastern European Medical Journal: SEEMEDJ, 4(1), 63-73. srce.hr
• Nambiar, A. K., Arlandis, S., B0, K., Cobussen-Boekhorst, H., Costantini, E., de Heide, M., ... & Harding, C. K. (2022). European association of urology guidelines on the diagnosis and management of female non-neurogenic lower urinary tract symptoms. Part 1: diagnostics, overactive bladder, stress urinary incontinence, and mixed urinary incontinence. European Urology, 82(1), 49-59. abdn.ac.uk
• Shaw, C. & Wagg, A. (2021). Urinary and faecal incontinence in older adults. Medicine. [HTML].
• O'Connor, E., Nic an Riogh, A., Karavitakis, M., Monagas, S., & Nambiar, A. (2021). Diagnosis and non-surgical management of urinary incontinence- a literature review with recommendations for practice. International Journal of General Medicine, 4555-4565. tandfonline.com.
• Pérez Carvajal, G. J. (2023). Relaci6n entre ingesta de protefna de alto valor biol6gico y prevalencia de Sarcopenia en adultos mayores de un centro geriatrico de la provincia de Chimborazo .. espoch.edu.ec
• Sandoval Animas, G. E. (). Sarcopenia y malnutrici6n en personas mayores, una revisi6n

bibliografica actualizada. repositorio.xoc.uam.mx. uam.mx
• Petermann-Rocha, F., Balntzi, V., Gray, S. R., Lara, J., Ho, F. K., Pell, J. P., & Celis-Morales, C. (2022). Global prevalence of sarcopenia and severe sarcopenia: a systematic review and meta-analysis. Journal of cachexia, sarcopenia and muscle, 13(1), 86-99. wiley.com.
• Gao, Q., Mei, F., Shang, Y., Hu, K., Chen, F., Zhao, L., & Ma, B. (2021). Global prevalence of sarcopenic obesity in older adults: A systematic review and meta-analysis. Clinical Nutrition. researchgate.net
• Almohaisen, N., Gittins, M., Todd, C., Sremanakova, J., Sowerbutts, A. M., Aldossari, A., ... & Burden, S. (2022). Prevalence of undernutrition, frailty and sarcopenia in community-dwelling people aged 50 years and above: systematic review and meta-analysis. Nutrients, 14(8), 1537. mdpi.com
• Moretti, D., Fiorillo, P., Mogliani, M., Buncuga, M., & Fain, H. (2024). Assessment of sarcopenia and muscle strength-related bioimpedance parameters in the preoperative spinal surgery consultation. Nutrici6n Hospitalaria, 41(1), 145-151. isciii.es
• Loyola, W. A. S., Corrales, G. A. L., Ganz, F., Caro, H. G., & Probst, V. S. (2020). Sarcopenia, definition and diagnosis: do we need reference values for older adults in Latin America? Revista Chilena de Terapia Chilena de Terapia Ocupacional, 20(2), 259-267. researchgate.net
• Criollo Sanchez, J. I. (2024). Use of dynamometry in older adults to determine sarcopenia. Revisi6n narrativa. udla.edu.ec
• Acosta-Benito, M. & Martfn-Lesende, I. (2022). Frailty in primary care: Diagnosis and multidisciplinary management. Atenci6n Primaria. sciencedirect.com
• Barajas-Galindo, D. E., Arnaiz, E. G., Vicente, P. F., & Ballesteros-Pomar, M. D. (2021). Effects of physical exercise in the elderly with sarcopenia. A systematic review. Endocrinology, Diabetes and Nutrition, 68(3), 159-169. [HTML]
• Murri, M. (2021). Effects of kinesiotherapy on sarcopenia in the elderly. ugr.edu.ar
• Castro Ellis, A. & C6rdoba Granados, J. (). Beneficios no cardiovasculares del ejercicio ffsico en adultos mayores. kerwa.ucr.ac.cr. ucr.ac.cr
• Kaçmaz, H. Y., Doner, A., Kahraman, H., & Akin, S. (2023). Prevalence and factors associated with frailty in hospitalized elderly patients. Revista Clfnica Espafiola. unirioja.es
• Montesino, D. C., Reguera, I. P., Fernandez, O. R., Relova, M. R., & Valladares, W. C. (2022). Clinical and epidemiological characterization of disability in the older adult population. Interdisciplinary Rehabilitation/Rehabilitacion Interdisciplinaria, 2, 15-15. saludcyt.ar
• Raymundo, R. R., Marfa, C. C. R. R., Edith, M. E. D., & Ernesto, R. O. R. (). Alteraci6n de la velocidad de la marcha y del test de levantarse de la silla:L Inicio del sfrome de fragilidad en mujeres mayores institucionalizadas?. academia.edu. academia.edu
• Barillas Escobar, E. J. & Henrfquez Mezquita, M. E. (2021). Analisis de la aplicaci6n de la Escala de Fried en el diagnostico de fragilidad en el adulto mayor que consulta a la Clfnica Comunal San Antonio Abad de la Redues.edu.sv
• Martfnez, J. M. O., Martfnez, P. H., & Macfas, J. G. (2024). Frailty, sarcopenia and

osteoporosis. Medicina Clfnica. [HTML].
• L6pez, T. E. (2023). Construcci6n, disefio y validaci6n de un instrumento de evaluación6n sobre el conocimiento del sfrome de fragilidad en adultos mayores. uaq.mx
• Fernandez, A. M., Reyes, M. J., & L6pez, M. I. V. (2022). Information and communication technologies (ICT) in training and teaching. FMC- Formaci6n Médica Continuada en Atenci6n Primaria, 29(3), 28-38. [HTML] [HTML
• Sanchez, I. V. M. D. O., Bravo, M. G. E., Reyes, A. T. C., Marfn, H. J. V., & Chacha, A. G. O. (2023). EduTrends: Navigating the Digital Age of Education. Editorial Investigativa Latinoamericana (SciELa). google.com
• Céspedes-Tamayo, L. G., Augello-Dfaz, S. L., & Ulloa-Cedefio, H. A. (2020). Social networks in the teaching-learning process. XIII Jornada de Aprendizaje en Red. researchgate.net
• Chaby, L., Benamara, A., Pino, M., Prigent, E., Ravenet, B., Martin, J. C., ... & Chetouani, M. (2022). Embodied virtual patients as a simulation-based framework for training clinician-patient communication skills: An overview of their use in psychiatric and geriatric care. Frontiers in Virtual Reality, 3, 827312. frontiersin.org.
• Siew, A. L., Wong, J. W., & Chan, E. Y. (2021). Effectiveness of simulated patients in geriatric education: A scoping review. Nurse Education Today. [HTML].
• Masud, T., Ogliari, G., Lunt, E., Blundell, A., Gordon, A. L., Roller- Wirnsberger, R., ... & Stuck, A. E. (2022). A scoping review of the changing landscape of geriatric medicine in undergraduate medical education: curricula, topics and teaching methods. European geriatric medicine, 13(3), 513-528. springer.com.
• Ong, E. Y., Bower, K. J., & Ng, L. (2021). Geriatric educational interventions for physicians training in non-geriatric specialties: a scoping review. Journal of Graduate Medical Education, 13(5), 654-665. allenpress.com.
• Wu, S., Jackson, N., Larson, S., & Ward, K. T. (2020). Teaching Geriatrics and Transitions of Care to Internal Medicine Resident Physicians. Geriatrics. mdpi.com
• Pan, F., Ge, L., Hu, M., Liu, M., & Jiang, W. (2024). Application of virtual diagnosis and treatment combined with medical record teaching method in standardized training of general practitioner. Medicine. lww.com
• Stefanowicz-Kocol, A., Grochowska, A., & Kolpa, M. (2023). A Model of Culture-Sensitive Blended/Distance Simulation Teaching and Learning in the Field of Geriatrics. atar.edu.pl
• Piot, M. A., Dechartres, A., Attoe, C., Jollant, F., Lemogne, C., Layat Burn, C., & Falissard, B. (2020). Simulation in psychiatry for medical doctors: a systematic review and meta-analysis. Medical education, 54(8), 696-708. sorbonne-universite.fr

# CHAPTER 4
# DIDACTIC SEQUENCES FOR TEACHING GERIATRIC SYNDROMES TO PHYSICIANS RESIDENTS

## Introduction

Population ageing is a global phenomenon that poses significant challenges and unique opportunities for the field of medicine. As the proportion of older adults in society increases, so does the prevalence of specific geriatric syndromes that require specialised care and careful management. Among these, frailty, sarcopenia, cognitive impairment, caesthesia, and urinary incontinence stand out as critical conditions that considerably impact the quality of life of the elderly. These syndromes not only affect the physical and mental health of individuals, but also impose significant burdens on caregivers, health systems and society at large. Recognising the growing need for effective and specialised training in geriatrics, this book is designed specifically for teachers who are at the forefront of medical education. Our aim is to provide a comprehensive guide to teaching geriatric syndromes, using a blended learning or B-learning approach, which combines traditional teaching methods with modern digital technologies. This methodology not only enriches the learning experience, but also allows for greater flexibility, accessibility and adaptability, essential elements for educating a new generation of doctors capable of meeting the challenges of geriatric medicine with competence and compassion.This chapter provides a series of detailed teaching sequences covering each of the major geriatric syndromes. These sequences are designed to make it easier for teachers to plan and implement effective courses by providing clear structures, recommended educational resources, practical activities, and methods of assessment. By integrating theory and practice, and by providing numerous examples of how to apply knowledge in real-life clinical situations, we hope to foster meaningful and lasting learning.By providing this comprehensive guide, we aim to support educators in their efforts to prepare future physicians by equipping them with the skills and knowledge necessary to improve the care and well-being of the elderly population. We firmly believe that quality medical education is the cornerstone for achieving exceptional geriatric care and responding effectively to the needs of an ageing population.

## 1. Detailed Didactic Sequence for Immobility Syndrome

Objective: To deepen the understanding of the causes, consequences, diagnosis and management of immobility in geriatric patients, focusing on evidence-based interventions and the implementation of personalised care plans.

### a. Theoretical introduction (Lecture and video)

Content: To provide a sound theoretical basis on what immobility is, its most frequent causes in the elderly population (neurological, musculoskeletal diseases, etc.), and the associated complications such as pressure ulcers, muscular atrophy, and psychological problems such as depression.

Resources:

- Reading: Articles and text chapters on epidemiology and pathophysiology of immobility.
- Video: Presentations by experts discussing cases and exploring the latest research on the topic.

Activity:

**b. Online discussion**

Discussion forum on the learning platform where students can ask questions, share clinical experiences and discuss best practices to prevent immobility.

Topics for discussion:

Strategies for identifying patients at risk, effective preventive measures in different care settings, and the importance of interdisciplinary work.

**c. Case study**

Description: Case analysis of an elderly patient with severe immobility due to a combination of severe arthritis and stroke. Students will assess the patient, identify potential problems and develop a management plan.

Activities:

- Functional assessment using standardised tools such as the Barthel Scale.
- Design of a rehabilitation plan including physiotherapy, nutritional interventions and psychosocial support.

**d. Virtual simulation**

Objective: To use simulations on the B-learning platform to practice physical assessment, differential diagnosis and implementation of a multidisciplinary management plan.

Simulated scenarios:

- Practice the management of a patient who has developed immobility after hip surgery.
- Interventions to prevent immobility in a patient with multiple comorbidities.

Methods:

**e. Evaluation**

- Interactive quiz: Multiple choice and true/false questions to assess the theoretical knowledge acquired about immobility.

- Personal reflection: A reflective report where the learner will discuss a continuous improvement plan based on a case scenario provided, reflecting on how they will apply the knowledge and skills learnt in a real clinical environment.

**f.Additional resources**

- Access to current research articles, so that students can keep up to date with the latest developments in the treatment and management of immobility.
- Webinars and conferences: Links to online conferences with experts in geriatrics and rehabilitation to expand your learning and understand different perspectives and approaches.

**2. Detailed Didactic Sequence for Falling Syndrome**

Objective: To train resident physicians to identify risk factors for heart disease, effectively assess patients at risk, and apply preventive strategies and effective treatments in the geriatric population.

a. **Interactive presentation (Webinar)**

Content: Introduction to the epidemiology of caudaemia in the elderly, both intrinsic and extrinsic risk factors, and the latest clinical practice guidelines for the prevention of caudaemia.

Resources:

- Webinar: Live presentation by a geriatric expert who will also address residents' questions in real time.
- Interactive Slides: Presentations that students can review at their own pace, with links to key studies and additional resources.

**b. Virtual workshop**

Activity: Practical sessions where residents learn to use coffee risk assessment tools such as the Tinetti Scale, the Lift and Walk Test, and other measures of balance and mobility.

Simulation: Use of virtual clinical cases to practice assessing patients, interpreting results and making decisions about appropriate interventions.

**c. Group discussion**

Description: Small group discussions using videoconferencing platforms to explore and discuss different preventive strategies adapted to various settings (such as hospital, home or long-stay institutions).

Objectives: Each group should develop a coffee prevention plan, taking into account the specific characteristics of the environment and the patient.

**d. Role-playing (Simulation)**

Aim: To practise interventions in controlled scenarios with actors or simulators representing elderly patients at high risk of coffee.

Activities: Implementation of preventive interventions, use of assistive devices, and how to educate patients and carers on the prevention of falls.

Methods:

**e. Evaluation**

- Practical skills test: Assessment of acquired competencies through a circuit of stations where residents demonstrate their skills in assessing and managing waterfall risks.
- Theoretical knowledge test: Online test including multiple-choice, true/false and short answer questions on the theory of coffee prevention.

**f.Additional resources**

Access to advanced simulations: A platform that offers more complex virtual scenarios for residents to practice identifying and dealing with coffee in a variety of situations.

Further reading and videos: Materials addressing case studies, reviews of effective interventions and new technologies in the prevention of cathaesthesia.

**3. Detailed Didactic Sequence for Urinary Incontinence**

Objective: To deepen the understanding, diagnosis and management of urinary incontinence in the geriatric population, promoting an integrated and multidisciplinary approach to treatment.

**a. Seminar**

Content: Overview of urinary incontinence, including classification of the different types (stress, urge, mixed, and overflow), and review of current treatment options.

Resources:

- Videoconference: Presentation by a specialist in urology or geriatrics explaining the physiological basis and clinical implications of incontinence.
- Articles: Assigned readings covering recent studies and updated clinical practice guidelines.

**b. Collaborative work**

Activity: In small groups, residents will develop an interdisciplinary care plan for a case study of a geriatric patient with urinary incontinence, taking into account medical, psychological, and social aspects.

Objectives: To integrate theoretical knowledge with clinical practice, encouraging collaboration between disciplines such as urology, nursing, physiotherapy and social work.

**c. Clinical simulation**

Description: Practical exercises on simulation platforms that allow residents to perform diagnostic assessments (such as medical histories, stress tests, and cystograms), prescribe treatments and manage follow-ups.

Activities: Simulation of patient interactions and clinical decisions based on test results and responses to previous treatments.

**d. Discussion Forum**

Objective: To facilitate a space for the exchange of experiences and strategies on the management of incontinence in different geriatric contexts.

Methodology: Facilitated discussions led by a moderator who poses clinical scenarios, ethical dilemmas and questions about treatment decisions, encouraging residents to contribute their opinions and prior learning.

Methods:

**e. Evaluation**

- Online exam: Test including multiple-choice questions, case studies and essay questions to assess theoretical knowledge and the ability to apply it in practice.
- Clinical case presentation: Residents will present a detailed analysis of a fictitious patient, including assessment, treatment options and follow-up plans, demonstrating their ability to integrate and apply acquired knowledge.

**f.Additional resources**

Learning platform: Ongoing access to a platform containing educational videos, interactive simulations and discussion forums to reinforce autonomous and continuous learning about urinary incontinence.

Webinars and workshops: Opportunities to participate in webinars and hands-on workshops on the latest innovations in the diagnosis and treatment of urinary incontinence.

## 4. Detailed Didactic Sequence for Cognitive Impairment

Objective: To equip resident physicians with critical skills and knowledge to assess, diagnose and manage cognitive impairment in the geriatric population, with a comprehensive approach that includes medical, psychological and social interventions.

### a. Online course

Content: A comprehensive introduction to types of cognitive impairment, including mild cognitive impairment (MCI) and various forms of dementia, such as Alzheimer's disease and vascular dementia.

Resources:

- Educational videos: Recorded presentations by experts in neurology and geriatrics, discussing the pathological basis and clinical manifestations of cognitive impairment.
- Digital readings: Articles and book chapters on the latest research and treatments available.

### b. Online discussion

Activity: Moderated discussion forums where residents analyse case studies to identify signs and symptoms of cognitive impairment, discuss assessment strategies and share management approaches. Objectives: To encourage critical reflection on diagnostic and therapeutic challenges and to improve residents' ability to work in an interdisciplinary team framework.

### c. Interactive activities

Description: Use of specialised software to conduct virtual cognitive assessments, including the Mini-Mental State Examination (MMSE) and the Montreal Cognitive Assessment (MoCA). Practice: Simulations that allow residents to apply these instruments in simulated clinical scenarios, followed by automatic feedback and detailed explanations of the correct answers.

### d. Study group

Activity: Regular study group meetings to review recent articles and discuss innovations in the treatment and management of cognitive impairment, including pharmacological and non-pharmacological therapies. Methodology: Small group analysis of recent literature, with group presentations summarising key findings and their clinical applicability.

Methods:

**e. Evaluation**

- Presentation of a management plan: Each resident presents a complete case, from the initial assessment to the management plan, including strategies for managing the medical, psychological and social aspects of care.
- Interactive test: An exam composed of multiple choice, short answer questions and case study scenarios to assess both theoretical knowledge and technical skills.

**f.Additional resources**

Access to conferences and webinars: Links to virtual conferences and webinars given by experts in cognitive impairment and dementia.

Lifelong learning tools: Subscriptions to neurology and geriatrics journals, and access to research databases to keep up to date on developments in the field.

**5. Detailed Teaching Sequence for Sarcopenia**

Objective: To provide resident physicians with the knowledge and practical skills to identify, prevent and treat sarcopenia in the geriatric population, using an integrated approach ranging from assessment to multidisciplinary intervention.

**a. Multimedia lessons**

Content: A detailed introduction to sarcopenia, including its definition, pathophysiological mechanisms, clinical impact and current diagnostic criteria according to the European consensus (EWGSOP2).

Resources:

- Educational videos: Presentations by geriatric and physiatric experts discussing the physiological aspects and consequences of sarcopenia.
- Articles and guides: Digital readings providing up-to-date information on the latest developments in sarcopenia research and treatment.

**b. Practical workshops**

Activity: Training sessions on how to implement physical exercise programmes and nutritional strategies to prevent and treat sarcopenia. Includes training in the use of resistance equipment and strength training techniques.

Methodology: Hands-on learning with live demonstrations and opportunities for residents to practice and receive direct feedback.

**c. Group discussion**

Objective: To analyse complex clinical cases to identify sarcopenia and discuss multidisciplinary intervention strategies.

Format: Facilitated small group discussions, supported by case studies reflecting different scenarios and levels of sarcopenia severity.

**d. Virtual laboratory**

Description: Interactive simulations in which residents use virtual diagnostic tools such as electrical bioimpedance and DEXA to measure body composition and diagnose sarcopenia.

Practice: Online exercises that allow residents to interpret test results and make clinical decisions based on simulated scenarios.

**e. Evaluation**

Methods:

- Practical and theoretical examination: Assessment of skills and knowledge acquired through an examination that includes both multiple-choice questions and a practical component, where residents must demonstrate their ability to assess and plan treatments for fictitious patients.
- Project presentation: Residents develop and present a comprehensive intervention plan for a case of sarcopenia, considering aspects such as exercise, nutrition and medical management.

**f. Additional resources**

Online webinars and workshops: Access to educational events featuring recent innovations and research studies on the treatment and management of sarcopenia.

Ongoing resource platform: Subscription to a platform offering regular updates, instructional videos and articles of interest on sarcopenia and geriatric health in general.

**6. Detailed Teaching Sequence for the**

**Frailty Syndrome in the Elderly**

Objective: To provide resident physicians with comprehensive training in the identification, assessment and management of frailty in older adults, integrating multidisciplinary approaches covering both prevention and intervention.

**a. Introductory Online Course**

Content: Fundamentals of frailty syndrome, including its definition, diagnostic criteria, and impact on the health and well-being of the elderly.

Resources:

- Educational Videos: Series of videos detailing the pathophysiology of frailty, associated risk factors, and clinical consequences.
- Recommended reading: Articles and book chapters on current models of frailty assessment and their clinical relevance.

**b. Interactive Workshops**

Activity: Practical workshops on how to use frailty assessment tools such as the Fried Frailty Scale and the Cumulative Frailty Index.

Methodology: Hands-on learning with case simulations, where residents apply these tools on simulated elderly patients, followed by group discussions on the results.

**c. Discussion Forums**

Objective: To discuss interdisciplinary management of frailty, sharing intervention strategies from different disciplines (medicine, nursing, physiotherapy, social work). Format: Online forums where residents can exchange ideas, discuss management strategies, and learn from the experiences of their colleagues and teachers.

**d. Case Management Simulations**

Description: Use of virtual clinical cases to practice decision-making in the management of frailty, including the planning of interventions such as exercise programmes, nutritional modifications, and psychosocial support.

Practical: Residents work in teams to develop integrated management plans, evaluating the effectiveness of different interventions through interactive simulations.

Methods:

**e. Evaluation**

- Practical assessment: Residents present their management plans through role-playing simulations, receiving real-time feedback on their clinical approach and communication skills.
- Knowledge test: A written test covering all theoretical aspects of frailty syndrome, ensuring understanding and ability to apply the knowledge acquired.

**f. Continuous Improvement Project**

Final activity: Development of a quality improvement project in a geriatric setting, where residents identify a frailty-related problem, analyse data, and implement an evidence-based improvement plan.

Objective: To apply the knowledge and skills acquired in a real-life context in order to improve patient outcomes in geriatric care settings.

**g. Additional resources**

Access to webinars and conferences: Links to conferences and webinars from geriatric experts discussing the latest advances and studies in the management of frailty.

Digital library: Ongoing access to a digital resource library with reading materials, instructional videos and best practice guides on frailty.

# CHAPTER 5
# USE OF ARTIFICIAL INTELLIGENCE IN GERIATRIC PRACTICE.

## Introduction

Population ageing is one of the most significant challenges facing global society in the 21st century. In Latin America, this demographic trend has become an undeniable reality, where the increase in life expectancy and the decrease in birth rates have resulted in a steady growth of the elderly population. According to data from the Economic Commission for Latin America and the Caribbean (ECLAC), by 2024, more than 15% of the total population of Latin America is expected to be 65 years of age or older. This demographic change poses significant challenges for the health care, quality of life and well-being of this growing population of older adults.

In this context, technology, and in particular Artificial Intelligence (AI), has emerged as a promising tool to address the challenges and needs of geriatric healthcare. AI has the potential to radically transform medical practice by offering innovative and personalised solutions that can improve the quality of life of older people, optimise resource management in the healthcare system and support healthcare professionals in clinical decision-making.

As we move towards a future where healthcare for older adults plays a central role in the sustainable development of Latin America, it is essential to explore and understand the role of AI in this context. This research aims to shed light on the challenges and opportunities that AI presents, thus contributing to the advancement of geriatric medicine in the region and the well-being of its senior citizens.

## 1. Artificial Intelligence Applied To The Geriatric Care

### a. Definition of Artificial Intelligence

Artificial intelligence (AI) is a rapidly emerging field in educational technology, including in the context of medical education (Zawacki-Richter O ;et al, 2019). AI, driven by machine learning algorithms, is gaining popularity in the healthcare sector and has the potential to improve patient care, real-time data analysis and continuous patient monitoring (Kolachalama, V. and Garg, P. , 2018) (Sapci, A. and Sapci, H. , 2020).

AI refers to the development of systems and algorithms capable of performing tasks that normally require human intelligence, such as natural language processing, machine learning and decision making.

### b. A.I. in Medical Education.

In the field of medical education, AI has diverse applications, such as personalised learning, data analysis, medical image recognition, and treatment plan decision making (Chan, K. and Zary, N., 2019) (Xu, H: et al, 2022). However, the adoption of AI in medical education faces challenges, including the need for educators to be more involved in AI research and implementation (Zawacki-Richter O ;et al, 2019).The integration of AI into medical school curricula is already being explored, and applications of AI technology are being felt in a variety of medical disciplines (Wood, E; et al, 2021). There is growing recognition of the potential of AI in medical education, including its ability to enhance teaching and learning processes (Popenici, S. and Kerr, S. , 2017). However, the adoption of AI in medical education requires careful consideration of factors such as curriculum revision, the inclusion of basic AI concepts in medical education, and the development of AI-enabled tools (Iqbal, S., 2022) (Memon, S;et al, 2021). The use of AI in medical education also raises ethical considerations and the need for bioethics education (Briganti, G. and Moine, O., 2020). As well as the impact of AI on the educational landscape and the psychology of the actors of the educational process (Dziatkovskii, A., 2023) and the knowledge and attitudes of medical students and educators towards AI in medical education (Doumat, G;et al, 2022).A key aspect of AI in the context of medical education is its ability to provide personalised and adaptive solutions. In this sense, it is important to recognise that the incorporation of artificial intelligence in the medical area, from the professional and academic dimension, is not intended to replace human work or knowledge, but rather to support medical practice and provide the necessary learning tools to the subject, facilitating its understanding during the training process (Aguilar Bucheli, D; et al, 2023).Machine learning (ML) algorithms, a branch of AI, are gaining popularity in the healthcare sector. AI powered by machine learning algorithms has the potential to transform medical education by providing personalised learning experiences and improving diagnostic accuracy (Kolachalama, V. B. & Garg, P. S., 2018). Artificial intelligence (AI) has shown enormous potential to transform the delivery and accessibility of healthcare in Latin America. The use of AI in this context can improve the health and well-being of older adults, assist in nursing care and address challenges related to medication adherence and disease management ( Garcfa Alonso R; et al, 2022).

### c. Situation of AI in Latin America

In Latin America, health systems vary from one country to another and find their major application benchmark in the field of cancer care (Garcfa Alonso R; et al, 2022) (Liliana, Sussman; et al, 2022); AI has become important in cancer care, with promising results in the prediction of clinically relevant parameters, cancer diagnosis, research and personalised medicine. However, development and cooperation in AI research and geriatric care in Latin America is limited.Strengthening collaboration and communication between countries, regions and institutions can further boost the development of AI in geriatric care in Latin America [3].Among the themes and areas of study in our region we can cite:Improving Health Care for the Elderly: The use of AI has an impact on improving patient safety in health care. This includes the detection early detection of diseases such as dementia and other geriatric problems, identification of adverse drug reactions during hospitalisation, and the creation of drug reconciliation lists to reduce clinical errors and improve ageing (Jehath Syed, 2022).Opportunities for Gerontological Nursing Practice: It has been discussed how AI can advance gerontological nursing practice, although specific details of the study were not available, it highlights the importance of AI in the health of older adults and its potential to improve gerontological practice (O'Connor S, 2022). Review of the Use of AI in Elder Care: A review study covers several types of AI technologies used in elder care, such as robots, ex-skeletal devices, smart homes, smart health apps and voice-activated devices. These technologies play roles as rehabilitation therapists, emotional supports, social facilitators, supervisors and cognitive promoters. The impact of AI on elderly care is promising, although more research is needed to validate these roles (Ma, B. et al, 2023).

Impact of AI on the Health of the Elderly and Potential Discrimination: The World Health Organisation has highlighted the ability of AI to predict health risks and personalise health care management. However, it also warns of the risk of age discrimination due to biases in the data that feed these technologies and in the design of the technologies. Policies have been proposed to ensure that AI has a positive impact on the lives of the elderly and that age discrimination is avoided (UN, 2022).

Balancing Safety and Autonomy for Older Adults: A workshop explored AI in the context of balancing safety and autonomy for older adults and people with disabilities. This approach underscores the importance of AI in helping these populations live as independently as possible (Lustig, T. A., & Cilio, C. M., 2019).

AI in the Care of Elderly People Living Alone: A study in Spain demonstrates how AI can help in the care of elderly people living alone, allowing family caregivers to monitor through a mobile application. This approach increases the safety and well-being of the family member and also includes remote companionship services and technical assistance (Infogeriatria, 2022). The relevance of this research lies in the imperative need to explore the characteristics of the application of virtual technologies by artificial intelligence in geriatric and gerontological care in Latin America. The relevance of this study lies in the urgent need to understand how AI is being implemented and used in geriatric medical practice in the Latin American context in the year 2024. Through a positivist approach and an exploratory design, this study aims to shed light on the following questions:

1. Evaluation of the adoption and use of AI technologies in elderly care in Latin America.

2. Identification of the advantages and challenges associated with the integration of AI into geriatric medical practice in the region.

3. Analysis of the potential impacts of AI on the quality of life of older adults and on the efficiency of health care services.

4. Evaluation of the perspectives and attitudes of geriatric health professionals towards AI as a complementary tool in their practice.

5. Identification of possible recommendations for the improvement of the implementation and adoption of AI in geriatric health care in Latin America.

In this sense, it is proposed to carry out an exploratory study to establish the basis for future research, in relation to the characteristics of the use of artificial intelligence in geriatric medical practice in the member countries of COMLAT (Latin American Committee of Geriatrics).

Garcia Alonso's (2022) study (Garcfa Alonso R; et al, 2022) concludes that: Artificial intelligence (AI) has the potential to transform the delivery and accessibility of healthcare in Latin America, particularly in low- and middle-income countries.

Artificial intelligence is also used for predictive analytics in healthcare, which helps identify patients at risk of developing certain conditions or complications. This can aid early intervention and personalised treatment plans.

Artificial intelligence-enabled chatbots and virtual assistants are used to provide basic health information and support to patients, helping to improve access to health services.

AI is being used for drug discovery and development, helping to speed up the process of identifying potential new drugs and treatments. Artificial intelligence is used for remote patient monitoring, allowing healthcare providers to remotely monitor patients' vital signs and health status, enabling timely interventions and reducing the need for face-to-face visits.

The study by Jingjing Wang, 2023 (Wang J, et al, 2023) "Application of artificial intelligence in geriatric care: bibliometric analysis" analyses current research hotspots and collaborative networks in the application of AI in geriatric care through bibliometric analysis.

The study revealed that research on the application of AI in geriatric care has developed rapidly, with a significant increase in publications between 2014 and 2022, accounting for 90.87% of all publications.

The main research hotspots identified in this field include Alzheimer's disease, care of the elderly, acceptance and monitoring and treatment of diseases.

Machine learning, deep learning and rehabilitation have recently become critical points of research on the application of AI in geriatric care.

The United States and the International Journal of Social Robotics have been the main contributors in terms of the number of publications on this topic.

**2. Considerations Ethical considerations**

Privacy and transparency issues in the use of patient data and records, as well as technological and regulatory difficulties, are challenges faced by Latin American countries in implementing artificial intelligence-based services in healthcare. The provision of artificial intelligence-based health services in Latin America contributes to promoting the United Nations Sustainable Development Goals (Garcfa Alonso R; et al, 2022).

## REFERENCES


• Garcfa Alonso R; et al. (2022). Digital Health and Artificial Intelligence: Advancing Healthcare Provision in Latin America. IT Professional. doi:doi: 10.1109/mitp.2022.3143530

• Aguilar Bucheli, D; et al. (2023). Artificial intelligence in medical education Latin Americancontext..Metro Ciencia, https://doi.org/10.47464/metrociencia/vol31/2/2023/21-34.

• Briganti, G. and Moine, O. (2020). Artificial intelligence in medicine: today and tomorrow.. Frontiers inMedicine, 7, https://doi.org/10.3389/fmed.2020.00027.

• Chan, K. and Zary, N. (2019). Applications and challenges of implementing artificial intelligence in medical education: integrative review. . Jmir Medical Education, https://doi.org/10.2196/13930.

• Doumat, G;et al. (2022). Knowledge and attitudes of medical students in lebanon toward artificial intelligence: a national survey study. Frontiers in Artificial Intelligence, https://doi.org/10.3389/frai.2022.1015418.

• Dziatkovskii, A. (2023). The ergonomic effect of AI & ML in education. https://doi.org/10.46916/26042023-1-978-5-00174-960-8.

• Infogeriatrics (2022). Retrieved 01 02 02 2023, from Infogeriatria: https://www.infogeriatria.com/noticias/20220113/estudio-demuestra-artificial-intelligence-helps-care-for-the-elderly-living-alone

• Iqbal, S. (2022). Are medical educators primed to adopt artificial intelligence in healthcare system and medical education?. Health Professions Educator Journal, 7-8. doi:https://doi.org/10.53708/hpej.v5i1.1707

• Jehath Syed (2022). Retrieved 02 02 2024, from s4be.cochrane.org: https://s4be.cochrane.org/blog/2022/10/14/involving-artificial-intelligence-technologies-in-the-care-of-older-people-the-future-of- healthcare/

• Kolachalama, V. and Garg, P. (2018). Machine learning and medical education.

. NPJ Digital Medicine, https://doi.org/10.1038/s41746-018-0061-1.

• Kolachalama, V. B. & Garg, P. S. (2018). Machine learning and medical education. , 1(1). . NPJ Digital Medicine, https://doi.org/10.1038/s41746- 018-0061-1.

• Liliana, Sussman. et al. (2022). Integration of artificial intelligence and precision oncology in Latin America. Frontiers in medical technology. doi:doi: 10.3389/fmedt.2022.1007822

• Lustig, T. A., & Cilio, C. M. (2019). Artificial Intelligence Applications for Older Adults and People with Disabilities: Balancing Safety and Autonomy: Proceedings of a Workshop-in Brief. (E. a. National Academies of Sciences, D. o. Education, H. a. Division, B. o. Services, B. o. Policy, & D. a. Forum on Aging, Edits.) National Academies Press (US). doi:DOI: 10.17226/25427

• Ma, B. et al. (2023). Artificial intelligence in elderly healthcare: A scoping review. Ageing research reviews. doi:https://doi.org/10.1016/j.arr.2022.101808

• Memon, S;et al. (2021). Perception about artificial intelligence in medical education. PJMHS,419-420.doi: https://doi.org/10.53350/pjmhs2023173419
• O'Connor S. (2022). Artificial Intelligence for Older Adult Health: Opportunities for Advancing Gerontological Nursing Practice. Journal of gerontological nursing, 48(12), 3-5. doi:https://doi.org/10.3928/00989134-20221107-01
• UN. (2022). Retrieved 01 02 2023, from UN News: https://news.un.org/es/story/2022/02/1503842
• Popenici, S. and Kerr, S. (2017). Exploring the impact of artificial intelligence on teaching and learning in higher education. . Research and Practice in Technology Enhanced Learning, https://doi.org/10.1186/s41039-017-0062- 8.
• Sapci, A. and Sapci, H. (2020). Artificial intelligence education and tools for medical and health informatics students: systematic review. . Jmir Medical Education, https://doi.org/10.2196/19285.
• Wang J, et al. (2023). Application of Artificial Intelligence in Geriatric Care Bibliometric Analysis. J Med. doi:DOI: 10.2196/46014
• Wood, E; et al. (2021). Are we ready to integrate artificial intelligence literacy into medical school curriculum: students and faculty survey. . Journal of Medical Education and CurricularDevelopment, https://doi.org/10.1177/23821205211024078.
• Xu, H: et al. (2022). Cultivation path of compound talents in ophthalmic diagnosis, treatment, and nursing based on artificial intelligence. Journal of Clinical and Nursing Research, 106-111. doi:https://doi.org/10.26689/jcnr.v6i5.4387.
• Zawacki-Richter O ;et al. (2019). Systematic review of research on artificial intelligence applications in higher education - where are the educators? International Journal of Educational Technology in Higher Education, https://doi.org/10.1186/s41239-019-0171-0.

## INDEX

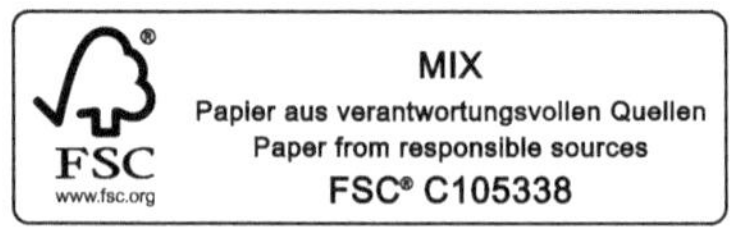


Printed by Books on Demand GmbH, Norderstedt / Germany